5 minute HEALTH BOOSTERS

CONSULTANTS
Dr Vince Forte BA MB BS MRCGP MSc DA
Fiona Hunter BSc Hons (Nutrition) Dip. Dietetics

5minute HEALTH BOOSTERS

How to sneak age-defying, disease-fighting habits into your life without really trying

Published by Reader's Digest Association Ltd
London • New York • Sydney • Montreal

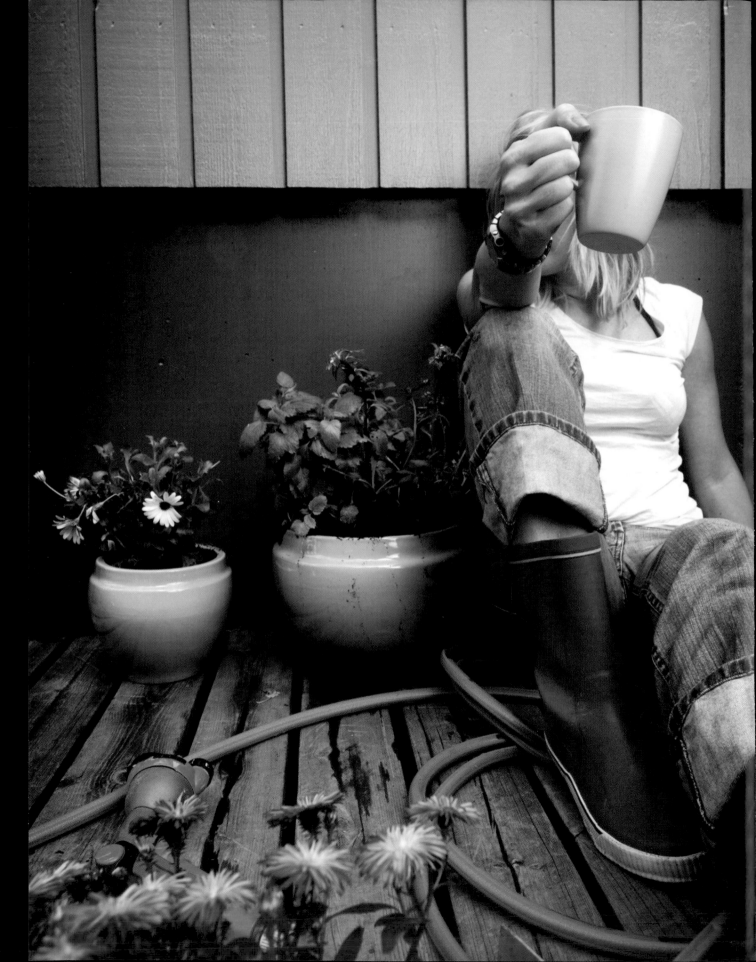

Introduction

Better living, without big changes

Everyone knows the old proverb 'prevention is better than cure' – but it's not always the easiest advice to put into practice. All the things you're supposed to do to prevent disease seem to require a lot of effort – and that in itself is enough to put you off trying. It's also difficult to see immediate benefits - prevention's reward is that a disease does *not* appear, so how will you know if it's effective? Combine the two problems and it's easy to see why people are often so reluctant to take active steps to ward off ill health.

The *5 Minute Health Boosters* team has tackled this head-on by reviewing hundreds of valuable acts of disease prevention and health promotion. The book explains how they work and the evidence that backs them up, and offers quick and easy ways to put them into practice and reap the benefits.

The result? Health promotion in tiny acts you can fit into your life, every day. Each tip is about one thing: improving the quality of your life, and the quality of your health.

As a full-time GP advising on preventative medicine every day, I know this approach makes sense, and that even the smallest act of health promotion is worthwhile. This book is about prevention you can practise on a daily basis. It's not about making room for health with laborious add-on effort: it's about finding room for prevention in the nooks and crannies of your life as it is right now.

Healthy living is something everyone can enjoy. With every bit of advice you act on in this book, the scales of health and happiness will tip ever further in your favour as *5 Minute Health Boosters* provides the elusive bridge to transport you from merely accepting the way you are living to leading a life you can love and cherish, in good health, for many years to come.

I am pleased and proud to recommend this book as an effective tool for reshaping your future health, putting control of your well-being and your own destiny firmly into your own hands.

Dr Vince Forte BA MB BS MRCGP MSc DA

Contents

part 1   THROUGH THE DAY   14–75

part 2   HEALTH BOOSTING COOKING   76–113

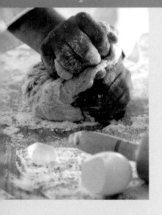

part 3   DINING OUT   114–131

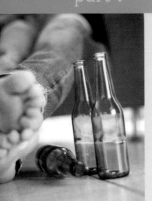

part 7 HABIT CONTROL 304–319

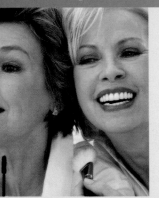

part 8 HEALTH BOOSTING LOOKS 320–339

part 9 PEOPLE AND PLACES 340–371

NOTE TO READERS While the creators of this work have made every effort to be as accurate and up to date as possible, medical and pharmacological knowledge is constantly changing. Readers are recommended to consult a qualified medical specialist for individual advice. The writers, researchers, editors and publishers of this work cannot be held liable for any errors and omissions, or actions that may be taken as a consequence of information contained within this work.

What are 5 MINUTE HEALTH BOOSTERS?

Small changes that quickly add up

Pick up any health or diet book these days and you come away with two impressions. First, it would appear that very few of us lead healthy lives and, secondly, there's a lot that needs to be corrected. On top of that, there's only one way to correct things – the hard way: with a complete lifestyle overhaul. Take, for example, a number of popular weight-loss programmes, which start with frightening 'induction phases' that involve a complete change in the way you eat, including the banning of whole categories of popular foods. The discomfort and discipline involved are on a par with military boot camp – which is exactly how some popular fitness programmes bill themselves.

Desire something a little more gentle? Pilates and yoga are terrific, but to reap the maximum benefits they require lessons, teachers and practice. And woe betide us if a GP discovers something wrong with our bodies – the regimen of pills, tests, diets and scary talk about healthy living can often seem worse than the problem itself.

But what if there were another way – a way to get the benefits of a lifestyle overhaul without the top-to-bottom revamping? An easier way. A way of making tiny change after tiny change (so tiny you barely notice you're making them), yet emerging in the end with the kind of major transformation that dramatically improves your health? That wouldn't be so bad and might really deserve some serious consideration.

Welcome to *5 Minute Health Boosters*, which redefines health as you know it. Living life the health-boosting way means choosing the raisin bran, not the toast and marmalade. It's taking a 5 minute walk when you're bored with your computer, rather than eating a chocolate bar. It's laughing when someone does something stupid, instead of shouting. It's going to sleep instead of watching the late film. It's snacking on a peach, not a cake. It's kissing your partner instead of walking out the door with only a goodbye.

After all, what is health, anyway? As defined here, health includes feeling relaxed rather than stressed; loving rather than getting irritated. It's finding time for yourself and your priorities that you didn't think you had. And, of course, it's also about healthier, glowing skin and steady, sustainable weight control. It's having more energy in the afternoon and evening, less likelihood of developing diabetes and heart disease, measurably lower cholesterol and blood pressure levels, higher self-esteem, a greater sense of personal safety and an enhanced ability to handle things without falling apart.

Health is about feeling good today and the probability of being well tomorrow. And that's not an either/or – but both. It's about taking good care of your body, mind and soul.

Easy changes

5 Minute Health Boosters is the ultimate guide to the little decisions we make that add up to an enormous influence on our health. It contains more than 2,000 choices and tweaks that you can make to your day, some so small as to seem almost inconsequential, yet guaranteed to make you healthier. The ideas are fresh, unusual, simple and fast. Best of all, they work.

And they're designed for the way you live your life. For instance, you're not being told to give up all salt. Instead, you'll find two dozen ways to reduce the amount of salt in your diet incrementally, until, ever so slowly, almost without noticing, you find that your salt intake has reached healthy levels – and your blood pressure has dropped as a result.

No time to exercise because you spend too much time driving? Find out how to combine the two. Too stressed to sleep, and too sleep-deprived to handle stress? There are dozens of simple remedies for both. Unhappy about overeating,

down to context. For example, coffee is great for you if your goal is mental sharpness and alertness. But for a good night's sleep, coffee is nothing but trouble. So try not to be confused by any occasional conflicts; instead, make choices that are most sensible for your particular goals.

A lifetime journey

The biggest problem with intense, highly defined health programmes is that they end – perhaps after as little as two weeks, or maybe as long as six months. And when they end, you're back to your old ways. Which is why our obesity

Health isn't merely the absence of disease. You're not healthy if you're perpetually stressed, frustrated or dissatisfied.

and overeating because you're unhappy? Learn some easy tactics that work during even the most frenetic days to improve your mood and control your appetite.

There may be times when you'll ask yourself, 'How can this advice possibly help my health?' It's a legitimate question. When you encounter tips that seem pretty far removed from the topic of health, such as how to organise your day or do chores more efficiently, the chances are they're about achieving calm or a positive attitude.

There are two reasons why they're here. First, health isn't merely the absence of disease. It involves mental and spiritual aspects as well. You're not healthy if you're perpetually stressed, frustrated or dissatisfied. Second, your mental and spiritual health have a direct link to your physical health. Research confirms it over and over. Stress, anger and other hostile emotions and attitudes are significant risk factors for everything from heart disease to obesity.

So even if some of the advice doesn't seem to have a direct health benefit, be assured that it does help. And remember that every tip in this book has come from a doctor or is doctor-approved.

Finally, you may find the occasional piece of advice that seems to contradict what's been said in a different place. In each case, it all comes

rates continue to rise, despite the many millions of pounds spent on weight-loss books and programmes. And why heart disease, diabetes and stroke – all lifestyle-influenced diseases – are rampant.

You'll find that the pursuit of better health has a momentum all of its own – when you do it the right way. One health-promoting habit will reinforce others. The chances are, after you've hit the threshold of making subtle, little adjustments to your lifestyle, you will, in fact, have introduced the sweeping improvements in your health that once seemed so elusive and intimidating. In other words, take enough small steps, one at a time, and you've accomplished the equivalent of reaching Everest's peak or circling the globe – without even getting out of breath.

5 Minute Health Boosters is the road map for your journey. It's the directions that enable you to take one small step, followed by more small steps, to introduce health promotion into the nooks and crannies of your life.

The bottom line: improving your health doesn't have to be difficult. In fact, it's mostly about common sense. Pick three health-boosting tips to do a day, every day, and you'll be well on your way to a lighter, more attractive, more disease-resistant and more contented you.

The everyday
HEALTH PLAN

Just say 'THREE A DAY'!

As with any programme designed to overhaul your health, *5 Minute Health Boosters* could seem overwhelming. After all, there are more than 2,000 tips on improving everything from the way you look to how much you weigh to your heart-health measurements to your relationships with loved ones.

Don't worry. The last thing this book does is overwhelm you – for that would be stressful and quite contrary to the book's optimistic, health-boosting philosophy.

So here's the proposal: every day, make three good-health choices that are outside your regular routine. That's all. Just three.

For instance, have a cup of tea instead of coffee in the morning. Substitute a bottle of water for your afternoon can of cola. Spend 5 minutes stretching in the morning while you watch the news. That's three. Call it a day. You'll do three more tomorrow.

Go ahead and make the same choices for tomorrow if you wish. But here's the one and only rule in this programme: once you've followed a choice for four days in a row, it no longer counts as one of your three choices. Instead, you should consider it a habit. It's time to add to it with a new and different good-health choice.

While you will recognise that habits are formed over months, not days, you also know that limiting yourself to three simple changes for weeks on end won't add up to much in the long run. Your goal is to sample new health tips, slowly and steadily. If they feel right, integrate them into your daily routine – again, slowly, steadily, over the days, weeks and months. Given time, you'll find that nearly every aspect of your life has changed in healthier ways – without you even noticing it!

That's it: the entirety of the everyday health plan. Make three healthy choices every day. With more than 2,000 to choose from in these pages, that should be easy.

The best tips for you

Just as there is only one rule to the programme, there's only one bit of expert advice to get you going: focus your efforts on the areas where you need the most help. For instance, if your major health concern right now is weight, choose three from the chapters that focus on healthy eating and weight loss. Having trouble sleeping? Three tips from the sleep chapter on page 72 should guarantee you a peaceful night's slumber. Which three? You choose. In all cases, it's your choice. For the book focuses on the idea that getting and staying healthy is an option and an opportunity, not an obligation. So you decide – as long as you do something, you've taken a small step towards better health. And through an accumulation of these small steps, you will reach your goal.

As you add three more healthy choices each day, the cumulative effect will be substantial. The outcome: a sustainable, healthy lifestyle marked by fewer colds, greater energy, a leaner, more attractive body, a happier outlook and greater resistance to chronic disease.

The health-boosting
PROMISE

Benefits that are proven and substantial

So just what is the health-boosting promise? Well, to start with, here's what it's not. It's not a promise that you'll lose 10lb in two weeks. Nor is it a guarantee that living the health-boosting way will provide you with boundless energy until a painless death, during your sleep, at the age of 107. But here's what medical studies suggest a health-boosting lifestyle *can* provide:

● **A leaner, healthier body for the rest of your life.** Of course, fad diets may kick-start your weight loss, but, as many of us have found out the hard way, in practice they're nearly always impossible to sustain over a lifetime. Instead, *5 Minute Health Boosters'* weight-loss tips are based on studies which show over and over again that the best way to lose weight and, most importantly, maintain the loss is simply through moderate daily exercise and healthy eating. Plus, there are some lesser-known research-based tips. Such as eating in front of a mirror. Cutting out soft drinks. Wearing blue while you're eating. All of these tips will help you to eat less and/or lose weight.

● **Better control of your blood sugar levels.** Just a brisk half-hour walk every day, or skipping sugary soft drinks and juices, or switching to whole grains, can decrease your risk of developing diabetes regardless of your weight.

● **A healthier heart.** It doesn't take much. One study found that a mere 30 minutes of walking three or more days a week could slash your risk of heart disease by more than a third.

● **Better control of your cholesterol levels.** Simply changing your eating habits from two large meals to six small meals a day, switching over to olive oil in your salad dressings, sipping

Special advice

There are more than 2,000 pieces of health advice in this book, all of them proven, valid, quick and effective. Of course, it's asking too much to suggest you consider each and every one. So, to help, certain tips are marked for quick spotting. These are the tips that you might wish to consider first, and they are identified as follows:

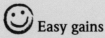

Fast results
These are tips that deliver benefits particularly quickly – in some cases, immediately.

Easy gains
These are health boosters that offer the best value for the least amount of effort.

Super-effective
This is advice that scientific research or widespread usage by experts has shown to be especially effective.

a cup of tea every few hours throughout the day, and sprinkling cinnamon on your cereal can significantly improve your blood sugar levels and reduce your risk of diabetes. Yes, it's that simple!

● **Stronger bones.** Here's one easy way: tend your garden for a few hours a week. One major study found gardening to be one of the best activities you can do for maintaining healthy bones. When you've finished, sip a glass of icy mineral water instead of a fizzy drink – that's more bone protection in yet another research-proven, health-boosting manner.

● **More intense workouts.** No, you don't have to give up walking for running; but little things, such as working out to an up-tempo musical beat, or working out in a room without mirrors, can result in a more intense workout and leave you feeling better at the end.

● **Improved control over stress.** A trip to the Caribbean would help, but that's not practical for most of us. How about hugging your partner, calling a friend, buying yourself flowers and decorating the walls of your home with art? All are simple changes, yet they've all been found to reduce stress hormones in various studies.

● **Enhanced energy.** Researchers discovered that just taking a 20 minute nap, having a sprig of rosemary to sniff or having a brisk walk up and down the stairs can leave you feeling refreshed and energised.

● **Improved memory.** Studies also find that switching to whole grains, mixing blueberries into your morning cereal and attempting the Sunday crossword puzzle can all help to maintain and even improve your memory.

The everyday health plan's
TOP 10 TIPS

If you read this book from front to back, you'll probably see some tips repeated again and again. This is deliberate – certain lifestyle changes have numerous health benefits. In fact, some bring so many gains that they've earned a place in the Top 10 list. Do these 10 things, and you're guaranteed to see the health benefits.

1 Drink a cup of tea in the morning.

2 Walk for 30 minutes a day.

3 Quit smoking.

4 Have a small glass of wine most evenings.

5 Take 5 minutes a day, close your eyes in a quiet room, and practise deep breathing.

6 Talk to a friend – whether in person, on the phone or via email – every day.

7 Eat fish twice a week.

8 Take a multivitamin with minerals every morning if your diet isn't optimal.

9 Eat whole, natural foods rather than packaged or processed foods.

10 Get a good night's sleep.

See how easy – and yet how beneficial – health-boosting living can be? Now, if you're ready, turn the page and embark on the easiest, healthiest changes you'll ever make in your life.

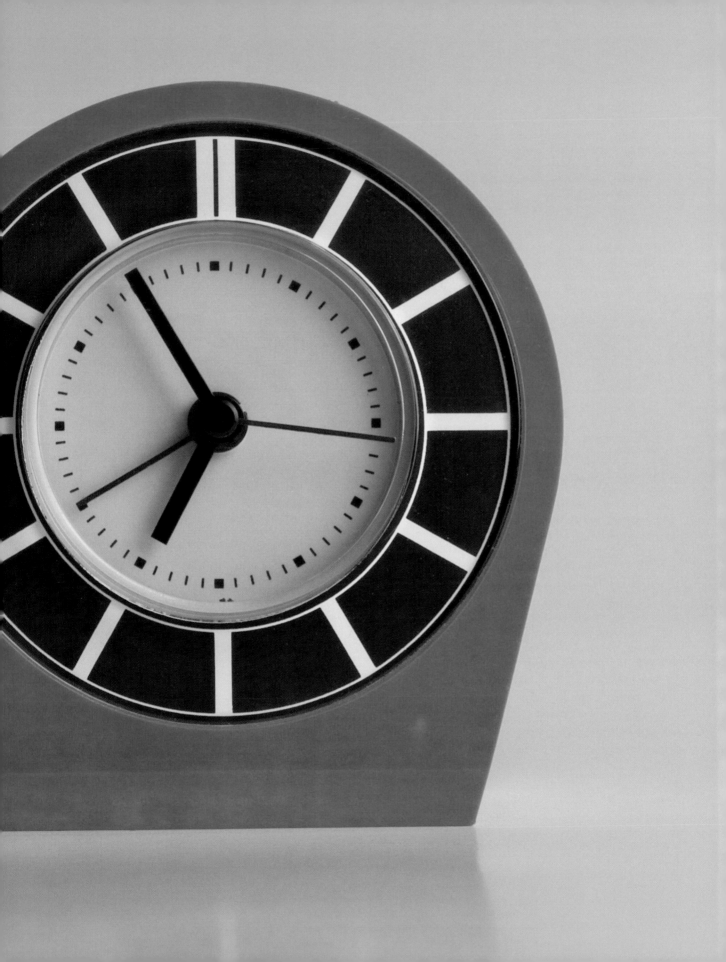

part 1

THROUGH THE DAY

From the morning shower to the evening news, your days are full of regular tasks and routines. Here's how to make each a little calmer, a little healthier.

The **WAKE-UP** routine

OK, it's probably no one's favourite time, particularly if you stayed up late the night before, but there are plenty of good reasons for starting each and every day as well as you possibly can. Here are some ways to make sure you get out of the right side of bed and ease yourself into things with a positive, calm attitude. Remember: stress and anxiety wreak havoc on your immune system. If you start out happy and relaxed, you greatly increase your chance of having a healthy, productive day.

19 WAYS TO BRIGHTEN UP YOUR MORNING

In winter, sleep with your blinds or curtains halfway open. That way, the natural light of the rising sun will send a signal to your brain to slow down its production of melatonin and bump up your levels of adrenaline, an indication that it's time to wake up. When the alarm goes off, you'll already be half awake. In summer, ensure your curtains are dark enough to keep out 5am sunlight, but leave your window open so you can wake to birdsong if you like to rise with the lark!

Set your alarm to go off 15 minutes earlier. That way, you don't have to jump out of bed and rush through your morning. You can begin the day instead by lying in bed, slowly waking up. Have a stretch, listen to the news headlines and mentally run through what you're going to wear, what you're going to do, what you're going to have for breakfast. It's just as important to prepare yourself mentally as well as physically for your day. These few minutes in bed, before anyone else is up, are all yours.

Stretch every extremity for 15 seconds. Try this even before you open your eyes. Lift your arm and begin by stretching each finger, then your hand, then your wrist, then your arm. Next, move on to the other arm. Then your toes, feet, ankles and legs. Finally, end with a neck and back stretch that propels you out of the bed. You've just limbered up your muscles and joints, and enhanced the flow of blood through your body, providing extra oxygen to all of your tissues.

Read a motivational quote every morning. This can provide a frame for the day, a sort of self-help talk that keeps you motivated, unlike the negative impact of the morning news. Another option: use a motivational mantra that provides a

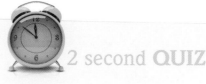
Mouthwash or toothpaste?
ANSWER: **TOOTHPASTE.**

Mouthwash will not keep your breath fresh for more than 20 or 30 minutes (tests with garlic revealed this), and most mouthwash contains alcohol, which can dry out your mouth.

meditation-like burst, or read or recite a poem that helps you to focus. A good one to use is Rudyard Kipling's 'If'.

Take a vitamin. If you have a well-balanced diet and are generally healthy, taking a multivitamin may offer no additional benefits, but if you are in the habit of skipping meals or are going through a period where you're not eating healthily, a daily multivitamin and mineral pill will ensure you get all the essential micronutrients your body needs. Think of it as a sort of insurance policy. Keeping a supply visible on the kitchen worktop will remind you to take one every morning.

Avoid any decisions. For truly relaxing mornings, reduce the number of choices and decisions you make to zero. Go about this in two ways: first, make your morning decisions the night before – what clothes to wear, what to have for breakfast, what route to take to work and so on. Second, make as much of your morning as routine as possible. Really, there's no need to vary your breakfast, timetable or bathroom ritual from one morning to the next.

Cuddle your children. Few things are more stressful in the morning than waking up an overtired seven-year-old

Healthy INVESTMENT

A sunrise alarm clock

You can find these intriguing alarm clocks in some electrical shops and department stores or buy them online. In addition to the typical radio/alarm, the clock can be set to become brighter gradually, as it gets closer to your wake-up time. The increasing light prompts your brain to begin making the stress hormone adrenaline, which helps you to wake up. You can also buy clocks that allow you to wake up to pre-recorded messages, to slowly building music coupled with an aromatherapy diffuser, or to an alarm that gradually increases in volume.

or a snoring teenager. Yet this is one of the few times when you can catch your children still vulnerable. Sit beside them and gently smooth their hair as you softly waken them, one by one. Or, if you're dealing with very young children, gently hug them awake. Such moments will send a quiet surge of joy through your entire day and will become all too rare in much too short a time.

Spend 5 to 10 minutes each morning listening to music or sitting just pondering. This allows the creative thinking that takes place during the night to gel and form into a plan of action, grounding you for the day.

Wake up to the smell of coffee. Buy the best coffee you can afford – fresh beans are best – and put twice the amount you've been using into your coffee-maker. Treat yourself to a machine with an alarm that can be set to start brewing at a specific time. The scent of strong coffee will pull you out of bed like a fish-hook in the back of your pyjamas. Morning is the best time to take caffeine – this central nervous system stimulant acts in many ways like other stimulant drugs such as amphetamines, waking you up and increasing your muscular activity. Even better: a study of 18 men found that caffeine improved their clear-headedness, happiness and calmness, as well as their ability to perform tests requiring them to pay attention, process information and solve problems.

Brush your tongue for 1 minute. There's no better way to rid yourself of morning breath and begin your day minty-fresh and clean. After all, more than 300 types of bacteria take up residence in your mouth every night. A quick brush over the teeth won't vanquish them all.

Drink a large glass of water. You've been fasting all night, so you wake up each morning dehydrated.

Fit in enough time to cuddle your children.

Check your morning calendar. First, hang a large calendar whiteboard in a prominent position in your kitchen. On it, write everything you need to know for that particular day, from the children's activities to whether someone is coming to service the boiler to whether it's time to pay the bills. Check it carefully while you sip that first cup of coffee or tea; it will help you to structure the day in your mind and avoid the stressful effects of forgetting something vital.

Create a checklist for your children. If you don't have children, skip this one. But if you do, to cut down on morning chaos, hang a whiteboard or blackboard in the hallway or kitchen and list all the things that must be done before the children can leave: brush teeth, eat breakfast, get schoolbag together, make bed and so on. Have them score through or erase each item once it's completed. You can do the same thing with lists printed out from your computer. Set a consequence: if all the items aren't ticked off 5 minutes before you need to leave, there's no TV/PlayStation/dessert/computer time that night.

Keep a wicker basket for yourself and each child by the front or back door. Into it go your keys, wallet and bag, along with the child's schoolbag, papers, gloves, hats, etc. This will prevent that frantic last-minute search for lost items.

Wash in a stress-free way. We spend an average of about 12 minutes in the shower. That's fine when you're preparing for a date, but in the morning you need to get in and out quickly. If you don't like showering the night before (it can do strange things to your hair!) try using two-in-one products such as a combination shampoo and conditioner.

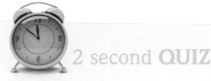

2 second **QUIZ**

Shower or bath?
ANSWER: SHOWER.

It's a healthier way to clean your body than soaking in the water you wash in. But baths are an excellent way to relax; for extra cleanliness use your shower attachment to rinse off afterwards.

When you wash your body, just hit the hot spots – your groin area and underarms. Everything else can just be rinsed off. The health benefit: reducing stress by saving time.

Prepare an emergency outfit in your cupboard. Include socks, jewellery, tights, etc., so on those mornings when you sleep through the alarm or simply need an extra 10 minutes, you can just pluck it off the hanger and go.

Dry more efficiently. Start with an oversized 100 per cent cotton bath sheet for maximum blotting. Towel-dry your hair and let it air-dry while you do your make-up or put on your underwear. Then, if you use a hair dryer, make it a high-energy one, at least 1,600 watts.

Hop on the treadmill for 30 minutes. Studies find that people who work out in the morning are more likely to stick to their exercise regimen because they get it out of the way first thing and don't have to come up with excuses later on. Plus, you'll produce endorphins whose mood-boosting effects will last most of the day.

Kiss all the people you love in your house before you leave, including pets if you like. Connecting with the ones you love soothes stress and helps you to focus on what's really important.

The **BREAKFAST** routine

There's a reason it's called the most important meal of the day. Not only is breakfast the first food and drink your body has had in more than 8 hours, but studies find that what you have for breakfast influences what you eat during the rest of the day. Additionally, people who eat breakfast are significantly less likely to be obese and have diabetes than those who don't. The most important tip is to have breakfast every day. Without exception. This one action alone can make a huge, positive difference to your health. But a doughnut or chocolate muffin won't do. The key is to choose energy-enhancing, health-invigorating foods. That's the focus of this part of the book.

23 WAYS TO KICK-START YOUR MORNING

✩ **Be consistent with your portions.** For most people, a perfect breakfast has three components: one serving of a whole-grain carbohydrate, one serving of a dairy or high-calcium food and one serving of fruit. Together, that would add up to roughly 300kcal. A high-protein serving (meat or an egg) is unnecessary but certainly acceptable, as long as it doesn't add too much fat or too many calories (more correctly, kilocalories – kcal – as you'll see on food labels) to the mix. Here are a few winning combinations, based on this formula:

● A bowl of high-fibre, multigrain cereal, with strawberries and low-fat milk on top.
● A cereal bar, an apple and a glass of cold milk.
● A pot of fat-free yoghurt with fresh blueberries mixed in, and a slice of wholemeal toast with a fruit spread.
● A mini wholemeal bagel, spread lightly with cream cheese and jam, and a peach plus a pot of yoghurt.
● A scrambled egg, a wholemeal roll, fresh-fruit salad and a cup of low-fat milk.
● A bowl of muesli or porridge with chopped banana or dried fruit.

☕ **Have a bowl of sweetened brown rice.** Consider this unique take on prepared cereal. Brown rice is full of energy-providing B vitamins, as well as being a great source of filling fibre. Cook the rice the night before, then, in the morning, put it in a bowl with a spoonful of honey, a handful of raisins, a cut-up apple and a sprinkle of cinnamon for a unique yet delicious treat. Don't like rice? Try other cooked grains instead, such as barley, oats, buckwheat, quinoa or millet.

✩ **Pour a cup of fruit smoothie.** Simply whizz a cup of strawberries and a banana in the blender, add a cup of crushed ice, and you've got a healthy, on-the-go

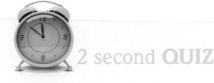
2 second QUIZ

Bacon or sausage?
ANSWER: **BACON.**

A slice of bacon, cooked thoroughly, has fewer calories than a typical sausage. Your best bet is a slice of lean back bacon with the rind and fat cut off, rather than fatty streaky bacon.

Orange juice counts as one of your five-a-day and may cut the risk of Alzheimer's.

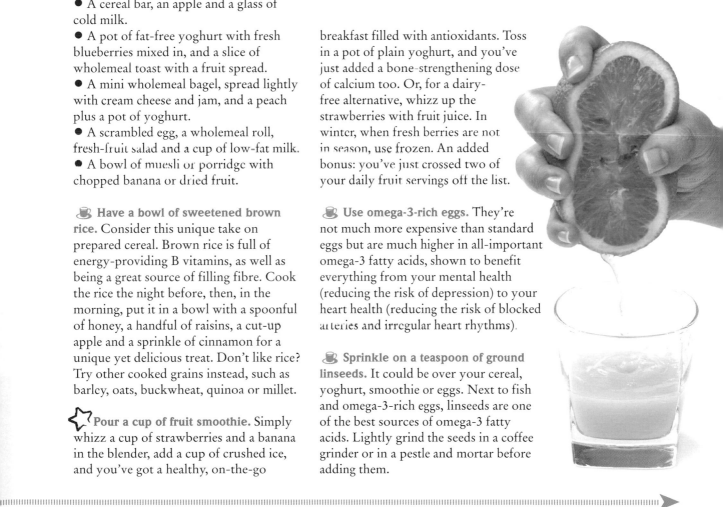

breakfast filled with antioxidants. Toss in a pot of plain yoghurt, and you've just added a bone-strengthening dose of calcium too. Or, for a dairy-free alternative, whizz up the strawberries with fruit juice. In winter, when fresh berries are not in season, use frozen. An added bonus: you've just crossed two of your daily fruit servings off the list.

☕ **Use omega-3-rich eggs.** They're not much more expensive than standard eggs but are much higher in all-important omega-3 fatty acids, shown to benefit everything from your mental health (reducing the risk of depression) to your heart health (reducing the risk of blocked arteries and irregular heart rhythms).

☕ **Sprinkle on a teaspoon of ground linseeds.** It could be over your cereal, yoghurt, smoothie or eggs. Next to fish and omega-3-rich eggs, linseeds are one of the best sources of omega-3 fatty acids. Lightly grind the seeds in a coffee grinder or in a pestle and mortar before adding them.

Healthy INVESTMENT

A blender
Why? Because blenders are great for making breakfast smoothies. You can toss in any kind of fruit – fresh, canned or frozen – along with fromage frais, quark or yoghurt for your calcium portion, a handful of nuts or seeds for heart-healthy fats, and a sprinkle of cinnamon for extra flavour. Add a glass of crushed ice in the summer for a cool drink, or warm it in the microwave for 30 seconds on cold winter mornings.

☺ **Use Flora pro.activ, Benecol or Danacol instead of butter.** These specially developed soft food spreads contain heart-healthy plant stanols. Just 2 tablespoons daily can significantly lower your total cholesterol level.

☕ **Make your own muesli.** Many shop-bought brands are filled with sugar and fat. To make your own, mix two parts porridge oats to one part dried fruit and seeds with a little brown sugar. Store in an airtight container. Not interested in do-it-yourself? There are a few shop-bought brands with reasonable sugar and fat levels – just read the labels carefully before you buy.

☕ **Eat half a grapefruit twice a week.** Grapefruit contains a good amount of folate and vitamin C, which are believed to help reduce the risk of heart disease and stroke. According to a review of eight studies in *The Lancet*, adding folic acid to your diet may cut your stroke risk by a fifth. But be cautious if you're taking regular medication. Grapefruit and its juice can interact with medicines that have to be processed through the liver, so check with your doctor first about any possible interactions between the grapefruit and any medication you're taking.

☺ **Sip a cup of green tea with your breakfast.** In addition to its heart-protective benefits, green tea may also have some weight-loss benefits, with one study finding that it appears to raise the rate at which you burn calories and increase the speed at which your body uses fat.

☕ **Top your cereal with soya milk.** Packed with potent phyto-oestrogens, soya has been credited with everything from protecting your heart to promoting stronger bones. But make sure that it's fortified with calcium for even more of the bone-building stuff.

☕ **Build your own breakfast and have great fun.** Who says breakfast has to be boring? Choose a selection of sliced fruit, yoghurt, whole-grain cereals and/or whole-grain toast, and let everyone mix and match to create their own toppings. If you're in a hurry, lay everything out on paper plates to make clearing up easier.

☕ **Add a vitamin.** If you are taking supplements, take them with breakfast, suggests nutrition expert Shari Lieberman, PhD, author of *The Real Vitamin & Mineral Book*. Taking supplements with food reduces the chance that they'll upset your stomach, as well as improving the absorption of minerals.

☕ **Spread apple slices with peanut butter.** The protein and fat in the peanut butter provide a good start to the day, while the apple and the quercetin it contains provide fibre and may protect against some cancers and heart disease.

☕ **Have a breakfast sandwich.** Top a wholemeal roll, bread or toast with melted low-fat cheese (low-fat mozzarella is a good choice), a sliced tomato and a sliced, hard-boiled egg.

☕ **Eat when you get to work.** If you really haven't got time or you simply can't face eating breakfast before you leave the house in the morning, keep a packet of cereal in your desk at work, or buy a low-fat sandwich on your way to work to eat when you arrive.

☕ **Visit the vegetarian section of the supermarket.** Veggie bacon, sausages and burgers are good sources of protein for breakfast without the saturated fat of their meat alternatives.

☕ **Sprinkle a handful of blueberries on your cereal.** Studies find the tiny purple berries are loaded with valuable antioxidants that can slow down brain ageing and protect your memory. Not into cereal? Try baking blueberries into oatmeal to create your own oatmeal and blueberry cereal bar, or mix them into wholemeal pancake batter.

☕ **Drink a glass of unsweetened orange juice every morning.** A small glass (150ml) of unsweetened fruit juice will count as one of your five-a-day. Plus, American researchers who followed almost 2,000 people for up to ten years found that the risk of developing Alzheimer's disease was 76 per cent lower in those who drank juice more than three times a week, compared to those who drank it less than once a week.

☕ **Eat a bowl of sliced strawberries three times a week.** Strawberries are packed with vitamin C and have numerous health benefits, one of them being protection for your eyes. One study of 247 women found that those taking vitamin C supplements were 75 per cent less likely to get cataracts than those who didn't take it. It's better, though, to get your vitamin C from food. Like other berries they're also rich in a wide variety of antioxidants, low in calories and even have a low glycaemic index (shown to keep blood sugar levels steady).

☕ **Slice two kiwi fruits into your morning smoothie.** You may have just reduced your risk of premature death by as much as 30 per cent. A British study found that every 30g of these vitamin C-rich fruits you eat a day reduces your risk of premature death by 10 per cent. Just slice the top off and scoop out.

☆ **Get at least 5g of fibre during breakfast each morning.** If you don't get off to a good start with your daily fibre intake, you'll never reach the recommended amount (24g per 1,000kcal). Plus, fibre is quite filling with no extra cost in calories. You can get 5g in just a few bites with a large raw apple, a small bowl of high-fibre cereal, 80g of blackberries or two slices of dark, whole-grain rye bread.

☕ **Choose these toppings for your (wholemeal) toast or bagel:**
● A tablespoon of low-fat soft cheese topped with a couple of tablespoons of mashed fresh raspberries or blueberries.
● One heaped teaspoon of peanut or almond butter.
● Mashed banana.
● One tablespoon of cottage cheese or low-fat soft cheese topped with a thin slice of smoked salmon.

☕ **Shave 30g of dark chocolate over a 250g pot of fat-free yoghurt, then mix.** The calcium-rich yoghurt can actually help you to lose weight, while the antioxidant-loaded dark chocolate can help to reduce the effects of 'bad' LDL cholesterol, keeping your arteries more flexible.

Add two vitamin C-rich kiwis to your morning smoothie.

The **PILL** routine

Between us, we take a lot of pills. The numbers may surprise you.

During any given week, around 80 per cent of us take some form of medication, according to NHS figures, with an estimated 834 million prescriptions filled or refilled in Britain in 2007, at a cost of roughly £10 billion. In addition, Britons spend £539 million on over-the-counter drug products a year. Not only that, a Food Standards Agency survey of almost 2,000 people in 2008 found that 36 per cent of us take a daily multivitamin.

Worryingly, one hospital audit found that 21.7 per cent of admissions among elderly people were the result of medication reactions, which suggests that too often we're taking our medicine incorrectly. By following these tips, you can make sure you take your drugs properly, avoid interactions and learn what to look for when buying over-the-counter drugs.

9 WAYS TO MANAGE YOUR MEDICINES AND SUPPLEMENTS BETTER

▶ **Each time you visit a new doctor, or revisit your existing doctor** after a period of several months, bring every pill you're currently taking with you. Simply put each prescription medicine, vitamin, herbal product, supplement and over-the-counter drug – even the aspirin – that you take in a typical day into a bag. Then ask your doctor to look over it all to see if there are any problematic combinations or if anything is redundant.

● **Ask your GP if there is a way to streamline** the medication you take. Some medicines can be taken once a day in sustained release, rather than three times a day. Others can be taken once a day or in a combination product that can decrease the numbers of drugs you're taking overall. Some can even be taken once a week.

● **Ask your doctor these questions about any new prescription:**
● What is this medicine for?
● What side effects might I encounter?
● What side effects are dangerous and should cause me to stop taking this medicine and call you?
● If I have to stop taking this medicine because of side effects, is there another that I can take instead?
● What are the dangers for me if I don't take this medicine?
● What time of day should I take it?
● Should I take it with food or without?
● Can I take it with any kind of liquid, or only with water?
● How will I know if it's working?
● How long should this medicine take to begin working?
● For how long should I continue taking this medicine?
Remember: while only a doctor can prescribe medicine, you are the one ultimately responsible for your health.

Choosing the
RIGHT VITAMIN

Been vitamin shopping lately? If you have, you probably needed a pain-reliever for the ensuing headache triggered by all those choices. Here's what clinical nutritionist Shari Lieberman, PhD, author of *The Real Vitamin & Mineral Book*, recommends to make it easier to pick the right ones:
● Choose natural versions, rather than chemically synthesised options, when buying fat-soluble vitamins, for example, A, D, E and beta carotene.
● Avoid additives such as coal tars, artificial colouring, preservatives, sugars, starch and other ingredients that you simply don't need with your vitamin.
● Don't bother about chelated minerals. Chelation means the minerals have an added protein to enhance absorption. But they're often more expensive, and studies that examine whether they really are absorbed faster than non-chelated minerals are sparse.
● Don't buy time-release formulations. These supplements may actually take longer to be absorbed and provide you with lower blood levels of the vitamin or mineral.

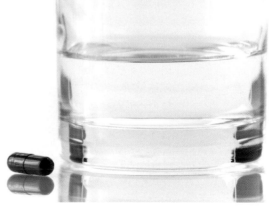

Get advice about how best to streamline your medicines.

Medicines for sale
OVER THE INTERNET

The internet has boosted sales of many over-the-counter drugs and supplements – and, more worryingly, prescription medicines, too. Since it's hard to know exactly whom or what you're dealing with in cyberspace, you need to take some special precautions.

- Check the validity of the pharmacy website. With the exception of getting discount deals on established over-the-counter medicines from truly recognised suppliers, such as major supermarkets and pharmacy chains, buying medicines over the internet is a risky business. There are a lot of fake medicines out there – the reason why the Royal Pharmaceutical Society of Great Britain (RPSGB) discourages buying prescription-only medicines online. They advise you to buy only from sites approved by the RPSGB, which will carry the internet Pharmacy Logo and carry an RPSGB membership number.
- Beware of purchasing drugs that aren't normally available in the UK. If in doubt, don't do it.

● **Get all your prescriptions at one chemist's or pharmacy,** and talk to the pharmacist. Pharmacists are more than just prescription fillers. They are specially trained in understanding possible medicine interactions, including interactions with herbal supplements. When you consolidate all your prescriptions, enlist your pharmacist's help to look out for these very things. In addition, some pharmacists receive special training in managing diseases such as hypertension and diabetes and can provide expert advice. They are also a great source of insider information on the most effective and best value over-the-counter drugs.

● **Then keep all your medicines in one place at home.** It is generally better to have everything together in one place rather than scattered around your house, car, bag or briefcase. Choose a space that is dark, and which is perpetually at room temperature (unless instructions call for medication to be refrigerated). It should be accessible to adults, but not children. While you are doing this, check each container to see if any has passed its expiry date. Throw out any prescription medicines you no longer need. Saving antibiotics for the next infection is the wrong thing to do.

☺ **Create a rigid pill-taking routine.** Aim to take your pills at the same time and place every day, and find a trigger to remind you to take them. Some pointers:

- Buy a pill box or other medication container and each Sunday evening re-stock it for the coming week. Place the pill box in a spot where you normally take your pills, and do not move it.
- Link your pill taking to a part of your morning ritual, such as brushing your teeth or drinking your first glass of water or juice of the day.
- Set the alarm on your watch, computer, mobile phone or personal organiser to beep when it's time to take a pill. Then, no matter where you are, or how busy you are, you'll get a reminder.

● **Watch out for shift work.** Working different shifts can create timing problems when taking your medication. Try to take them when you would normally have a shift change so the timing is similar whether you're going to bed or at work.

● **Buy measuring spoons just for your medicine,** and store them with your medicine. A kitchen teaspoon or tablespoon is rarely accurate.

☆ **Always follow the golden rules of medicine.** None of the following tips is particularly clever or surprising, but they all bear repeating – and adhering to:

- Disclose everything to your doctor and pharmacist: that you have allergies, that you are pregnant, that you have particularly high or low blood pressure, that you are prone to nausea, that you are on a diet. All are factors that can affect a drug's efficacy.
- When you collect your prescription, open the bag immediately to verify that the medication you received is the correct one, at the right dosage and for the correct duration.
- Ask your doctor or pharmacist if a medicine or supplement should be taken with or without meals.
- Take only the amount of medication prescribed or listed on the label.
- Get your prescriptions made up during slow times for the pharmacist, to avoid mix-ups.
- Whenever you purchase a supplement, ask your pharmacist if it has any potential interactions with any prescription or over-the-counter drugs you're taking.
- Don't use or share medication prescribed for someone else.
- Don't take your medicine in the dark or without glasses on or contact lenses in if you need to wear them.
- Keep your medicines in their original packaging with the full instructions; do so even for over-the-counter and herbal products.

Do **THREE** things...

Here are three useful pieces of advice on managing your medicines:

1 Find out from your pharmacist if the medication can be put into different containers such as a day-by-day pill box. Some medicines are light-sensitive or may not be compatible with plastic.

2 Try to fit in taking your medication with your daily routines. It's best to be able to associate your medication with a daily activity, such as washing your face.

3 Make a chart or have a pharmacist make a chart of each of your medicines and the times at which you take them. Put the chart on the fridge door.

Buy a pill box and keep it in a prominent place.

Reminder

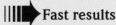 **Fast results**
These are tips that deliver benefits particularly quickly – in some cases, immediately.

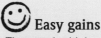 **Easy gains**
These are health boosters that offer the best value for the least amount of effort.

☆ **Super-effective**
This is advice that scientific research or widespread usage by experts has shown to be especially effective.

The COMMUTE

If you're like most people in Britain, it takes you about 45 minutes to get to work, more than anyone else in Europe. With the average daily distance travelled standing at 8.5 miles, this means that over the course of a year, you're spending about 360 hours and covering more than 4,000 miles – just getting to and from work! So it should come as no surprise that in one of the few major studies ever conducted on commuters, researcher Meni Koslowsky, PhD, a psychology professor from Bar-Ilan University in Israel, found that commuters experienced significantly high levels of tension. However, Dr Koslowsky also found that stress is not a forgone conclusion.

The tips that follow are designed to help you make your commute less of a strain, saving precious wear and tear on your heart, brain, immune system and emotions.

21 TIPS FOR A HAPPIER JOURNEY

● **If at all possible, use public transport.** Here's why. Dr Koslowsky's research found that it's not the commute per se that is so stressful. The real stress comes from the issue of control. If you drive your own car to work, part of the reason you do it is to feel that you're in control. So if you get stuck in traffic, you feel that you have lost control of your commuting experience, which is where the stress comes in. By taking public transport, be it the train or bus, you have already given up control of your commute. If you get stuck, you won't be blaming yourself for the delay. Nor will you be torturing yourself to solve the situation.

● **If it's a viable option, take the train.** Going back to that control issue again, Dr Koslowsky found that another major cause of commuter stress is uncertainty. And there is far more uncertainty in driving a car, or even commuting via bus or car-sharing because of traffic accidents, jams, etc., than in taking a train, as arrival times are more concrete.

● **Consider car-sharing.** It's not for everyone, and the research is ambiguous, but it is worth considering. On the one hand, Koslowsky's research finds that car-sharing can reduce stress, both in terms of the 'giving up' of control and in terms of the social interaction that occurs. But if you're an introvert who prefers a quiet commute so you can read, think or listen to music, then car-sharing with people who expect conversation could just stress you more. The bottom line: if you're an outgoing people-person, try the car-share. If you're an introvert, stick to your usual mode of transport.

● **Avoid rush hour, whenever you can.** It's such an obvious way to improve your commute, yet the fact that streets

2 second **QUIZ**

Manual or automatic?
ANSWER: **AUTOMATIC.**

The two main arguments for driving a manual car – you'll burn more calories and less petrol – don't hold up. Changing gears and using a clutch pedal don't add up to exercise unless you're driving an 18-wheel tractor. And on new cars, automatic transmissions have become increasingly fuel-efficient. From a stress point of view, an automatic will make driving much easier.

and trains are packed every rush hour shows that few people manage to find an alternative. What are the viable options, other than moving or getting a new job?
● Ask for a 1 hour shift in the time you start and end work.
● If your company has satellite offices that are closer to home, see if you can work there sometimes.
● Drive in before the crowds, and create a constructive pre-work ritual for yourself, such as exercising, eating a leisurely breakfast, running errands.

● **If you drive, take the route with the least stop-and-go traffic.** Longer is better if the traffic flows smoothly and you avoid lots of lights, roundabouts and zebra crossings. For most of us, no form of driving is as stressful as trying to move quickly on crowded main roads.

☺ **Above all, lose the 'race' mentality.** All that weaving, darting and surging rarely gains you more than a few minutes, but at a huge price to your stress levels (not to mention the extra wear and tear on your car and lower petrol mileage). Drive calmly, without abundant lane changes or speed surges, and your commute will become so much more pleasant.

● **Don't be judgmental about thy fellow driver.** It's a funny thing about high-stress drivers. When someone passes them, they get angry. When someone is going slower than they are, they get angry. They get angry when others forget to signal a turn, or if their car is larger or they're playing their music too loudly. Get over it! Overreacting to other drivers is a sure road to stress, headaches and anger. Instead, be a defensive driver, and never let what other drivers do bother you.

● **Learn while you commute.** If you've always been meaning to learn to speak Spanish or read the latest best-sellers, now's your chance. You can borrow audio books on CD from the library or download them from the internet to burn onto CDs or upload onto your MP3 player. Even coming to a standstill is bearable when you're in the thick of an exciting story.

● **Use your mobile phone for personal conversations only.** While mobile phones are definitely a boon to the commuter, Dr Koslowsky's research finds that using them for work-related tasks, such as setting up meetings, only increases your stress because it increases your working day. The best thing is to turn it off.

● **Leave 10 minutes earlier than you have to.** Do this both coming and going. Studies find that the less sense of 'time urgency', or worry about being late, you have, the less stressed out you'll feel during your commute.

● **Create a selection of music just for the commute:** one for going to work and one for relaxing on the way home from work. Workout experts know that music can serve many purposes and that each selection needs to be tailored to an individual's needs. Play the selection on an MP3 player if you take the train or bus or in the stereo of your car. Sing along if you're in your car. There's no need to be shy. The music has another benefit if you're driving: one study found that people who listened to music when stuck in a traffic jam were less likely to get angry and violent than those who didn't.

● **Practise good car ergonomics.** That means more than just buckling up. Before you head out, make sure your headrest is set directly behind your head, aligned with the top of your ears. Adjust your seat and steering wheel for maximum comfort. Check each mirror to make sure you don't need to lean or crane your neck to get the best vision. Now you can belt up.

● **Play a game.** Remember the old 'I Spy' games you used to play as a child on interminable trips? Invent your own version. Maybe you count the number of women you see applying make-up while driving. Or the number of people you see scratching their head. Start counting them each day and see if you can beat your previous day's record.

▐▐▐➡ **Equip your car.** Make sure you have the following with you: a spill-proof coffee cup filled with your favourite brew, a bottle of water and a bag of non-perishable snacks (try cereal bars and dried fruit) in case you get caught in traffic just as your blood sugar plummets. An audio book in the event of traffic coming to a complete halt and a fully charged mobile phone with headset will also come in handy.

● **Develop five alternative routes for your commute.** Again, this goes back to the control issue. If you know you can go a different way, you automatically have more control over the situation.

● **Prepare for your commute the evening before.** Check the weather, transport and traffic reports on local websites for information on possible hold-ups and delays. Listen to local radio for warnings and updates. Again, this puts the control back into your hands.

● **Relax before you begin your journey.** Instead of gulping down a scalding cup of coffee and choking down toast en route, get up early enough to enjoy a leisurely breakfast. Once you arrive at work, take another few minutes to sip a cup of tea or coffee before diving into your work. On the way home, go to the coffee area before you set out and just sit quietly with a drink for 5 minutes before heading home.

● **Work out in your car.** Do isometrics while driving by tensing and relaxing your leg muscles, tensing your arm muscles against the resistance of the steering wheel and/or tensing your abdominal and chest muscles. When done correctly for bouts of 10 to 15 seconds, these toning exercises can make an appreciable difference to your appearance, improve your fitness and relax you without distracting you or adding an extra minute to your schedule.

● **Lift your legs up and stretch them for 30 seconds.** This is one to do if you're on public transport or, if you're driving, when you've stopped in traffic. But this movement is important because it reduces the risk of blood clots from sitting too long in one position. Also put one arm behind your neck and stretch it by holding on to the elbow with the opposite arm. Switch sides. Do one every time the traffic comes to a halt.

● **Sniffed your car lately?** If you use your car as a mobile rubbish bin, you're putting more than your upholstery at

risk. Dirty cars can become a rolling Typhoid Mary, filled with insects, germs, mould, pollen and other irritants and pathogens destined to leave you sneezing, itching, watering and feeling sick. Even if you spend just an hour each day in your car, that's several times longer than most people spend in the bathroom!

● **Set your mood using the radio.** Tune into a music station and a news station. Use your travel time to catch up with the news, then switch to music before you arrive to relax or energise yourself.

In PERSPECTIVE

Why stress affects your health
You might think commuting has little to do with health, but the stress that comes from commuting almost certainly affects your well-being. Here's why.

Every time you're confronted with a stressor – whether it's a traffic jam, or something more serious, such as a fire – your body releases stress hormones such as adrenaline and cortisol. They, in turn, send signals to various parts of your body to ready them for action. For instance, your liver releases glucose to provide instant energy to muscle cells. Your lungs expand, your heart beats faster and your blood pressure rises to send more oxygen-rich blood throughout your body. All of this can lead to common stress-related conditions ranging from chronic hypertension, angina and gastric reflux, to constipation and irritable bowel syndrome, to depression, anxiety and fatigue.

Stress can even make you fat. Cortisol is not only a powerful appetite trigger; chronically high levels actually stimulate the fat cells in the abdomen to fill with more fat, creating a life-threatening form of fat called visceral fat, which puts you at higher risk of heart disease and diabetes.

Being tense can also inflict damage on your immune system. Like most body systems, it has a feedback loop. After the immune system has finished attacking foreign invaders, the brain sends out cortisol, to suppress the immune response. If your body is releasing cortisol all the time, as it does under chronic stress, then your immune system is constantly being suppressed, increasing your risk of illness.

Starting your
WORKING DAY

Have you ever been guilty of ending a bad day at work by snapping at the children, being rude to your partner, gorging on junk food, slumping in front of the TV or turning to alcohol? A bad work day may not seem unhealthy in itself, but it can serve as the domino that starts off a whole chain of destructive actions.

The way you begin your working day sets the tone for the rest of the day, not only in your workplace but also at home. A few simple measures taken at the start of your day can make all the difference to how it ends. Here are some tips to help you get off to the right – and healthy – start.

19 IDEAS FOR LAUNCHING A CALMER, MORE PRODUCTIVE DAY

▐▐▐▶ **Limit your work-starting routine to 15 minutes.** Don't spend more than a quarter of an hour getting coffee, settling in, looking at newspapers or reading emails. You are often at your freshest and most productive at the beginning of the day. A prolonged morning routine takes the positive edge off and makes your afternoon more stressful. Better to jump into the important work quickly, and read the non-essential emails after you've covered lots of ground.

◉ **Write two to-do lists.** The first should contain everything that you need to get done soon. It should be a comprehensive list of short, medium and long-term projects and work, and you should constantly adjust it. The second to-do list should be what you can reasonably expect to get done today, and today only. Be fair to yourself. Factor in the likely disruptions, meetings, phone calls and travel hassles. Make the tasks as specific as possible (for example, conduct online research for a particular market) and assign a time you plan to devote to it (20 minutes). Print the list out on brightly coloured paper; this keeps it from getting lost on your desk. By prioritising your work and breaking it down into small, achievable pieces, you greatly increase the chances that you will be satisfied with your day's accomplishments.

☆ **Take a few moments to assess the day's emotional challenges.** Almost as important as your to-do list is a 'be-prepared-for' list. Make an inventory of tough phone calls, boring meetings, challenging customers, frustrating red tape, infuriating rush-hour commutes, droning detail work and other mental challenges you are likely to face. Then accept that they are inevitable and prepare yourself to get through them

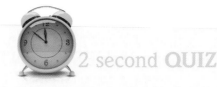

without anger, frustration or impatience. Remember: it's usually not work that gets us down, but rather the challenges that lie along the periphery of the job.

◉ **Visualise your day.** Taking that last point a little further, you might wish to start each day by closing your eyes for 10 to 20 seconds and visualising how you want it to go. See yourself making a stellar presentation at the board meeting. Experience the great feeling you're going to have when you finally make the sale or get that report off your desk. Hear yourself providing positive feedback to your employee, or even your boss. If you are religious, make this a prayer.

◉ **Schedule some social time for midmorning.** You probably work with people whom you like and know well. In fact, camaraderie is what makes many jobs great. So build a ritual into each morning in which you can spend a few moments of social time with colleagues. Make it short, at an appropriate time, and don't let a day go by without it. But avoid personal phone calls if you can; they can unexpectedly turn into big time-eaters.

◉ **Likewise, schedule some reading time.** There's not a job that doesn't require at least some reading, be it about the company, the industry, the marketplace, the economy. Create a ritual

WORKPLACE
madness

Most days of the week, you get up, get dressed, eat breakfast and head out into one of the unhealthiest places in the world. Problems at work are more strongly associated with health complaints than any other cause of stress – even more than financial or family problems. In fact, US researchers have found the first-ever link between stress and back pain. It turns out that people who get upset when they're criticised in the workplace use their muscles in ways that might lead to injury over time. Here is a wide spectrum of health-boosting tips to help you to cope with stress at work.

31 WAYS TO CALM THE CHAOS

☎ **Work on one thing at a time.** Today's office worker changes tasks an average of every 3 minutes. Such a lightning-speed day of interruptions is helped along by the multi-tasking made possible by computers. Working on eight things at once might seem impressive, but it isn't. Rather, it is exhausting, inefficient and highly stressful. So, instead of constantly checking emails, having two or three documents open on your screen, or returning emails as they come in, structure your day to focus on one thing at a time. In particular, start your day by blocking out 2 hours for uninterrupted hands-on work. During this time, do not answer your phone or check emails. Then check emails and respond all at once. Go to lunch. Structure your afternoon in the same way. Designate a time immediately after lunch and an hour before you leave for returning calls.

▐▐▐▶ **Work in short bursts.** The flip side to multi-tasking is that it is hard to sustain creativity or intensity on one task for long stretches. Rather, our brains work in cycles of creativity, then take a rest. So try this: after an hour or so of concentrated work, get up for 5 minutes, walk around, do some stretches. Not only will this help the quality of your work – by the time you finish your day, you'll have fitted in 30 minutes of stress-reducing exercise.

☎ **Deal directly, but constructively, with difficult workplace relationships.** 'Toxic people' are those whose negativity, intensity or demeanour always seems to drain or annoy you. This might be your boss, your assistant, your colleague – in other words, they are people with whom you frequently interact. After a negative encounter with a toxic person, the temptation is to be angry and accusatory. But that leads nowhere. Instead, try

Healthy INVESTMENT

An indoor water fountain
The sound and sight of running water can be very calming. Plus, a fountain on or near your desk acts as a humidifier amid the dry, overprocessed air of many offices. Small fountains are available to buy, while larger ones can be rented. Usually you just add water, plug it in and keep an eye on the water level as the days go by.

this direct, honest and disarming approach: 'I am finding our interactions stressful because of — — and am feeling bad about — —. I would like our working relationship to improve. What suggestions do you have for me?' Even if you feel that the other person is the one who should change, by asking for his or her suggestions, you avoid putting that person on the defensive. If your colleague is even a little bit reasonable, this might make him or her admit, 'Well, I suppose there are some changes I could make too.'

✩ **Praise yourself at least once a day.** Most of us don't take enough time to praise ourselves for doing things well. So when you've completed an interim or long-term goal, tell yourself – out loud – what a good job you've done. You'll get a burst of confidence that will go a long way towards helping you to maintain your cool amid the workplace madness.

☎ **Be creative in motivating yourself.** Here's a good one: write a cheque to an organisation you loathe, put it in a stamped, addressed envelope and tell a trusted friend to post it if you fail to meet an important deadline or complete a vital task. Or take the positive route: give the friend something you really cherish or desire and let your friend give it back to you only if you achieve your goal.

Shout or walk away?

ANSWER: **WALK AWAY.**

Shouting means the disagreement has become overly personal and emotional. Little good will come of it. Cut off the conversation firmly by saying this is an unacceptable way to resolve an issue and that you'll reconvene the discussion when your colleagues have regained their composure, thoughtfulness and perspective.

☎ **Forego the coffee during team meetings or group work.** A study sponsored by the British Economic and Social Research Council found that when men drank coffee while working together in a group, it tended to make the group less effective. The study also found that just the perception that the drink contained caffeine – whether or not it actually did – also increased the men's feelings of stress and their heart rates.

☎ **Stand against the wall and slide down it as if you were sitting** in a chair. Stay there for a few minutes without looking down, just feeling your spine against the wall. Breathe deeply (in through your nose, out through your mouth) and focus on one peaceful thought (waves crashing on the shore, a glass of wine by a roaring fire). Press your feet into the ground as you hold this position and picture the stress oozing out of your body. When you stand up, shake out your arms and legs and return to work refreshed.

☎ **Keep a holiday file on your desk.** Fill it with brochures of places you'd like to visit. When you're feeling stressed, daydream your way through it. It will remind you of one reason you're working, and provide a little virtual vacation.

☎ **Read a poem out loud twice a day.** The cadence, words and images will soothe your soul. Not into poetry? If you're religious, try reading a psalm or other sacred writings. If you love music, listen to a few of your favourite songs.

☎ **Make an altar or display in your office to remind you of your life** outside the office. Include pictures of your spouse, children and/or pet, a photograph of yourself doing something fun, plus a memento that reminds you of a special occasion. When you feel yourself getting overwhelmed and stressed out, take 5 minutes and simply stare at the display. Recall the day each picture was taken. Hold the memento and return in your mind to the place where you got it. Now you're ready to return to work.

☎ **Keep a work diary.** This is a diary you keep in your desk drawer (preferably locked). Write in it whenever you feel your temper rising, your frustration growing or your despair increasing. In it, you can write all the things you'd like to say to the boss/client/colleague so you get it out of your system without losing your job. It will also help you to understand what it is about your job and your day that really drives you crazy – and what you actually enjoy. Do not, however, keep said diary on your computer, and always, always keep it out of sight.

☎ **Take an impromptu holiday.** If you're experiencing an unusual number of headaches, a sore neck, sore back or other aches and pains; find you have trouble falling or staying asleep; or are snapping at your colleagues for no reason, it's time for a day off. Check your calendar for the coming week and find the first available day you can take. If you really are feeling unwell, take it as a sick day rather than a holiday - there's no shame in admitting that you are unwell. Whether you do something special or simply rest, make sure you take days off when you need them – if you don't you can bet you'll be really sick before the month's end.

☺ **Schedule 10 minutes of 'worry time'.** Close your office door or go and sit in an empty conference room and focus on what is stressing you out. You can bring your diary or just a sheet of paper. Divide the paper into three columns: My Worry; Why It Worries Me; Worst Thing That Could Happen. Once you confront the worst thing that could possibly happen – and realise that it's highly unlikely it ever will happen – you can get back to work with your worry load lightened.

☆ **Manage your email.** With about 5.5 trillion emails sent each year, an amount that increases by 40 per cent annually, this electronic form of communication has become a major source of stress. A study by the University of Western Ontario found that managers spend more than an hour a day on email, extending their working week by an average of 5 hours. The study also found that only 17 per cent of email users can answer their emails in the same day. To cope:
● Read emails once, answer immediately, delete if possible or move them to folders. Overflowing inboxes are depressing and take too long to read and sort.
● Insert email responses in the subject line whenever possible rather than composing a new message each time, and reply only when you have something to say.
● Use the automatic signature function in your email so that people can phone you or send you information via snail mail.
● Don't waste time acknowledging receipt of email. Also, don't email and phone with the same message.

Are you a WORKAHOLIC?

Sharon Lobel, PhD, professor of management at the Alber School of Business and Economics at Seattle University, has an interesting perspective on workaholism. Rather than saying that all workaholics have a problem, she divides them into two types: Happy Workaholics, who don't wish for a different lifestyle, and Unhappy Workaholics, who complain regularly.

'Happy Workaholics value work more than other aspects of life and arrange their lives accordingly,' she says. 'If people love to work and spend most of their waking hours at work, that's not a problem, in my opinion. On the other hand, if other people wish they had more time to devote to family, fitness or hobbies but are prevented from doing so because they work too many hours, those people are Unhappy Workaholics.' So how can you tell which category you fit into?

'People who say they're working to "advance in my job" or "to buy a house" are probably not Unhappy Workaholics,' says Dr Lobel. 'Unhappy Workaholics are likely to say their employer makes them work long hours and they're likely to express resentment towards the employer.' So what do you do if you find you're in this latter category?

'I think everyone needs to ask themselves what really matters in their lives,' says Dr Lobel. 'Which values are most important? Achievement, wealth, social justice, health, relationships? Then you need to look at how you're living your life. Do you devote time and energy towards what you most value? If the answer is yes, there isn't much of a problem. If the answer is no, it's time to implement some change.'

● Don't insert the recipient's address first before composing the email message. You might mistakenly send a message before it's finished or when it's saying something you didn't want it to say.
● Use the 'rule of three': if you've gone back and forth three times on a topic and you're still confused or have questions, pick up the phone.
● Never send an email if you're angry. You can write it (either as a draft, or preferably in your word-processing program) then save it and look over it when you feel calmer.

Listening to music in the office makes you more positive.

☎ **When things feel as if they're falling apart all around you, take 5 minutes and draw.** Seriously. Grab a pencil and some blank paper and sketch the chaos around you, or something funny, something peaceful or a caricature of the office villain. Using another part of your brain and focusing on something outside the chaos will provide a much-needed break.

☎ **Listen to music in your office.** A study by Sheffield University found that listening to music in an office-based working environment led to workers having a more positive mood, which they believe improved their overall work performance. One thing: it was important that the workers were able to choose the music themselves.

☎ **Talk to your best friend at work.** Studies find that social support at work is associated with lower blood pressure during the working day and smaller blood pressure surges even during work-related stressful moments.

☎ **Rub a drop of lavender oil on your inner wrist.** The aroma of lavender (or cucumber oil) is a known relaxant. Close your eyes, hold your wrist up to your nose and sniff deeply, picturing as you do a field of lavender in Provence, the purple stalks waving in the breeze.

☎ **Leave the office for lunch every day.** Getting out of the office, away from the stress and into a totally different environment, clears your mind and helps you to put some perspective on whatever hassles are dogging your day.

☎ **Build rewards into your working week.** Having something to look forward to makes every difficult task more bearable. It might be a special dinner, a film, a game of tennis or a massage. Put it in your schedule wherever it will help the most and think of working hard in advance to get to that reward.

☎ **Eat three Brazil nuts.** They're an excellent source of selenium, a mineral that may help to prevent depression.

☎ **Munch on a handful of pumpkin seeds.** A useful source of iron and micronutrients, these taste delicious and are a healthy way of providing a distraction from stressful moments in the working day.

▐▐▐▶ **Eat peppermint chocolates.** Treat yourself now and again to some peppermint chocolate – particularly good if it's dark chocolate. The chocolate itself is stress relieving, the peppermint provides a burst of minty energy and the tiny sugar rush might be just enough to get you over the hump. At the very least, it's better than slamming your office door or reacting in otherwise self-defeating ways to a madness-filled workplace.

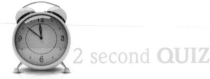

2 second **QUIZ**

Complain or keep quiet?
ANSWER: **COMPLAIN.**
Complain effectively, by being specific and positive, focusing on how correcting the problem will help the company and by providing at least one viable solution to the problem. Any sensible business wants to do things better. If your boss or company is so insecure or political that you can't speak honestly about things that need to be fixed, it's time to move on.

☎ **Pour a cup of boiling water over a handful of camomile leaves** or a camomile tea bag. The herbal mix, long known for its gentle, soothing properties, will help to de-stress and centre you.

☎ **Hold one nostril closed with a finger and blow strongly out** through the other (blow your nose first!). This is a yoga movement believed to reduce stress.

☎ **Walk and talk slower.** This tricks your body into thinking that things are calmer than they actually are.

☎ **Examine your real feelings.** If you love what you do, the stress related to your job will be far less damaging than if you don't. But if you hate your job, it's time to explore other options. Spending a few minutes each evening rewriting your CV and researching other job options or employers can help you to handle the stress at your current job.

☎ **Offer feedback.** As they say, it's better to give than to receive. Provide praise and recognition to others at work whenever it is appropriate. You will feel good by making others feel good, and the good feeling will tend to spread.

☎ **Have a 'perspective reminder' handy.** Work may seem overwhelmingly stressful at times, but your troubles are likely to be smaller than they seem. Keep a picture in your office – the earth taken from space, a starry night or the ocean – and look at it whenever you feel overwhelmed. Amid countless stars and the timeless crashing of waves against the shore, how important is that deadline, really?

☎ **Plan ahead.** When work is challenging, devote some of your down time – weekends and evenings – to delineating a

---

In PERSPECTIVE

Why is work so stressful?
There are lots of reasons. The experience is so widespread that the US National Institute for Occupational Safety and Health (NIOSH) has compiled a list:

● **How tasks are designed.** Heavy workloads, infrequent rest breaks, long working hours, shift work and hectic and routine tasks with little inherent meaning, and which don't use workers' skills, can all cause stress.

● **Management style.** If your workplace (or manager) discourages worker participation in decision making, micro-manages, has poor communications and lacks family-friendly policies, this is a potentially harmful environment.

● **Interpersonal relationships.** Do you get support and help from colleagues and supervisors, or do you feel as if you work in a pit of vipers? If the latter, it's a major stressor.

● **Work roles.** If you have conflicting or uncertain job expectations, get too much responsibility heaped upon your shoulders or feel you are wearing too many hats, you're working in a toxic waste dump when it comes to stress.

● **Career concerns.** Job insecurity, lack of opportunity for growth, advancement or promotion; rapid, unexpected changes; and continued rumours of redundancies and belt tightening can all land you with stress-related illness.

● **Environmental conditions.** Unpleasant or dangerous physical conditions such as crowding, noise or air pollution can turn any work environment into a stress pool.

---

sequence of tasks. Make a list, place boxes next to each item and tick off the boxes as you move through the list (which is in itself very satisfying). You'll avoid forgetting anything, you'll stay focused on the job, you'll be more efficient and it's very satisfying to tick off those boxes.

☎ **Socialise your work.** Suggest a once-a-week lunch gathering with colleagues where you can talk about a particular work issue. Use the collective brain to figure out how to do something better, improve your work facilities, perhaps, enhance productivity or improve relationships.

The **LUNCH** hour

For too many of us, the lunch break has become just another extension of our already overburdened day. Although the lunch hour was originally designed for just that – lunch – today we spend our time at midday running errands, pecking away at a computer keyboard or returning personal phone calls. When we do actually sit down to eat, it's often to consume whatever comfort food we can scrape together from the company vending machine or cafeteria. Yet your lunch hour offers the perfect time to break this hectic cycle. Rather than spending the time stressing over what you still need to accomplish or wolfing down fatty, salty, high-calorie foods, consider the following advice.

15 WAYS TO MAXIMISE YOUR MIDDAY BREAK

☺ **Go outside.** If you work in an office or a retail establishment, you're likely to be stuck in the same building all day long. Now's your chance to escape. Soak up the sun, watch the rain or feel the wind. Breathe some real air and disconnect for a moment from the job. At least once every day you should make the time to step outside, even if just for 2 minutes. It will recharge your body and mind.

● **Daydream for 15 minutes – then eat, run errands or return to work.** Creative daydreaming is not only a way to get out of the daily lunch-hour grind, but it's also a way to put your creative juices to work. If you're feeling particularly stressed about a project, spend your quarter of an hour exploring ways you can tackle it. If you feel mentally stale and burned out, spend the 15 minutes in la-la land, on a mini holiday. Imagine yourself strolling along the beach, climbing a mountain or generally spending time in a location that makes you happy.

● **Nap for 10 to 15 minutes.** Studies increasingly show the value of short naps during the day, and progressive employers are becoming more lenient about them. So if you can, curl up under your desk, nod off in your car (unless you're driving!) or otherwise arrange yourself in your office chair so you can snooze without anyone noticing. Your nap will refresh your mind and put a whole new perspective on the afternoon, because it breaks the tension of the day.

● **Pack a ready meal.** They're not just for dinner. You can pop your meal into your break room microwave for a quick-and-easy lunch that allows plenty of time to run errands or power walk during the rest of your lunch hour. Today's frozen food aisles include organic, vegetarian, low-fat, low-carbohydrate and numerous other healthy food options. Look for a frozen dinner that supplies fewer than 400kcal and less than 15g total fat, 5g saturated fat and 1.5g salt.

☆ **Practise the art of preparing a quick and healthy packed lunch.** Making your own lunch need not take a lot of time or creative energy. Include a source of lean protein, fruit or vegetables (raw carrots, celery, broccoli or cauliflower florets with a bit of low-fat salad dressing work well) and whole rather than processed grains. Leftovers from last night's dinner work wonders, as do the following quick-and-easy sandwich options:
● Peanut butter and banana sandwich: two slices of wholemeal bread topped with 2 tablespoons of peanut butter and half a sliced banana.
● Chicken or tuna salad sandwich: 170g of water-packed tuna or cooked chicken breast pieces mixed with 1 tablespoon of light mayonnaise and relish or grated carrots, served between two slices of wholemeal bread.
● A wholemeal pitta bread 'pizza': one pitta stuffed with low-fat pizza/spaghetti sauce or salsa, reduced-fat shredded mozzarella cheese, grated carrot, broccoli pieces, peppers, tomatoes, spinach, mushrooms or other veggies of your choice, plus lean ham or fat-free veggie sausage. Melt in the microwave before eating if desired.

Peanut butter and banana sandwiches – quick, easy and healthy.

2 second QUIZ

Lunch or graze?
ANSWER: **GRAZE.**

Nibble food throughout the day, rather than having a large, formal lunch. Spreading out your calories stabilises blood sugar and insulin levels, provides more frequent relief from stress, tension and boredom, and avoids the post-meal fatigue, because you don't have a big meal. Plus, you never get really hungry, and so are less likely to make the regrettable food choices that you might when you're starving. Best reason: all-day grazing frees up lunchtime for other things, such as a walk or catching up on work so you can get home a bit earlier and go for a walk then.

● Tortilla roll-up: 1 wholemeal tortilla spread with 1 tablespoon of low-fat soft cheese, topped with 2 slices of lean ham or wafer-thin sliced turkey and various veggies such as chillies, lettuce or spinach, tomatoes, onion, cucumber, sprouted seeds or grated carrots.
● Cheese and salad sandwich: 2 slices of wholemeal bread spread with 1 tablespoon of light mayonnaise or mustard and filled with 1 slice of low or reduced-fat cheese, along with lettuce, sprouted seeds and sliced avocado, tomatoes and peppers.

● **Pack ready-to-eat soup.** Your supermarket stocks numerous healthy soups sold in microwaveable cartons. One study suggests that broth-based soups help you to feel full, although they have few calories. Pack a bean and vegetable soup along with a couple of oatcakes spread with low-fat soft cheese and a carton of juice. With this easy lunch you'll have put together all the protein and fibre you need to power your body and brain through the afternoon.

● **Get away from your desk – even if it's just for 15 minutes.** No matter how pressing that big project is, physically remove yourself from your office for at least 15 minutes. Walk the corridors, chat with a friend or, as mentioned before, go outside. The time away from the desk will refresh your mind, allowing you to return to work more invigorated.

▮▮▮▶ **Make better menu choices.** If you have arranged a business lunch or lunch in a restaurant with friends or colleagues, try to be the first to order. Studies show that we're often swayed by other people's choices, so be sure you forge ahead by picking healthy options (see page 116).

● **Don't be tempted by meal deals.** When buying lunch, especially from fast-food restaurants, don't be tempted by any 'meal deal' unless it offers healthy options as part of the deal. Otherwise you may end up eating more than you actually want.

● **Create a sandwich chart and stick it on your fridge.** This prevents the early-morning haze from overcoming your better judgment and allowing you to leave the house without a packed lunch. In one category on your chart, list your bread options (wholemeal bread, pitta, tortilla wrap and so on). In the next column, list your protein options, such as turkey breast, low-fat cheese, lean roast beef, hummous or tuna/chicken salad. In another column, list vegetable toppings such as broccoli, bean sprouts, spinach, lettuce, cucumber slices, tomato slices, roasted red peppers and grated carrots. Finally, in the last column, list your condiments, ranging from mustard to low-fat mayonnaise to Italian dressing. You can also include a list of accompaniments such as cheese sticks, apples, oranges, yoghurt, baby carrots, low-fat milk and ready-made soup. Then, every morning (or, even better, the night before) pick one item from each column to pack. Voilà! A quick, healthy lunch.

● **For a healthier lunch, eat a healthier breakfast.** Breakfasts composed of simple starches such as pastries, white breads or many popular breakfast cereals are quickly converted into sugar that floods your bloodstream then goes away quickly. This leaves you craving fatty, high-calorie foods at lunchtime. Far better is to eat healthier breakfast foods that are digested slowly and thus leave you feeling fuller for longer. These include whole grains and lean proteins.

● **Walk to the sandwich bar.** If you must eat out, walk to your destination. You'll burn some extra calories and refresh your mind at the same time. The short walk may also give you the will-power you need to order more healthily.

● **Improve your work performance with healthy food.** Studies have shown that serving healthy food options and replacing fizzy drink-filled vending machines with machines filled with juice and water leads to pupils behaving better and achieving more in the classroom. The pupils were found to pay more attention and to be better able to focus

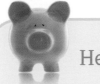

Healthy INVESTMENT

A small cooler and ice-packs
Ice-packs and coolers keep healthy food fresh until lunchtime, whether or not you have a fridge handy. An ice-pack or cooler will be particularly useful if you have a job that keeps you on the road.

on a task. And a British Food Standards Agency report, linking temper tantrums and bad behaviour in younger children on artificial food additives, has advised parents to avoid foods containing these additives. So why not follow the lead and switch to healthy, natural lunches to find out what it can do for your mental outlook and motivation.

● **Exercise as you run errands.** If you need to run errands during your lunch break, get in some exercise at the same time. If possible, power walk to the bank, shops, post office, etc. The exercise will help to refresh your mind and reduce the stress of the day.

● **Start a lunch bunch group.** Eat with other colleagues who are interested in weight control, health and nutrition. Share foods for taste-testing, exchange tips and recipes and once a week ask each member to bring in one healthy contribution to the meal.

Reminder

 Fast results
These are tips that deliver benefits particularly quickly – in some cases, immediately.

 **Easy gains**
These are health boosters that offer the best value for the least amount of effort.

☆ **Super-effective**
This is advice that scientific research or widespread usage by experts has shown to be especially effective.

Afternoon
DOLDRUMS

If you're like many people, shortly after lunch your head begins buzzing, your concentration plummets, your eyes droop and the top of your desk begins to look as cosy as a feather mattress. There are many plausible theories for the midday dips: the morning surge of hormones has petered out; some degree of 'brain tedium' – in other words, boredom – has set in. Or it may have something to do with what you ate; all meals divert blood from your brain to your gut but some foods also bump up levels of the soporific hormone serotonin. While the midday doldrums are common, they're not inevitable, especially not if you follow these tips.

20 IDEAS TO BOOST YOUR SPIRITS AND YOUR ENERGY

Before and during lunch…

● **Head outside and sit in the daylight for 10 minutes.** Better still, have your lunch outside and divide your break between eating and a walk. Here's why: your office probably has about 500 luxes of light, which is equal to about 500 candles. That compares with 10,000 luxes at sunrise and 100,000 at noon on a July day. So when the afternoon doldrums hit, go outside and sit in the sunlight. It will help reset your chronological clock, keep down the amount of melatonin (the sleep hormone) your body produces during this circadian dip and give you a valuable boost of beneficial vitamin D, reducing your risk of osteoporosis as well as various cancers.

● **Take a brief midmorning break for tea, coffee and/or a snack.** Use this time to relax and refocus, but, more importantly, to consume a few calories you might otherwise eat at lunchtime. Shrink the size of your lunch accordingly and the result will be less stupefying later.

☺ **Snack all day long.** Simply snack on nutritious foods whenever you get hungry, rather than eating lunch per se but watch portion sizes. Then use your lunch break for some kind of exercise, whether it's in the company gym or walking around a park.

☆ **Choose activating protein not energy-sapping carbs.** So a tuna salad without the bread is a better choice than a tuna sandwich. A green salad sprinkled with low-fat cheese, a hard-boiled egg and some sliced turkey wins over a pasta salad. The change can really make a difference. When researchers compared men who ate a 1,000kcal lunch with those who ate a 300kcal lunch or skipped the meal altogether, they found that when given a chance to nap after lunch, nearly all of the participants did so. But while the lunch-eaters slept for an average of 90 minutes, those who skipped lunch slept for only 30 minutes. These were also high-carbohydrate lunches (carbs stimulate serotonin release, which increases sleepiness), which may have contributed to the napping. You shouldn't skip lunch altogether, but the combination of eating less and eating fewer carbohydrates should lead to less sleepiness.

After lunch…

● **Enjoy teatime.** Get into the routine of a midafternoon cuppa. It's a good step towards beating the afternoon doldrums thanks to that little bit of a caffeine burst and the few quiet minutes it entails. The aim is not to munch down scones and clotted cream, but you can do better than a tea bag dunked in your unwashed coffee mug. Keep a selection of exotic flavoured teas (preferably caffeinated) in your office and an aesthetically pleasing cup just for tea. When the doldrums hit, brew yourself a cup and sit somewhere quiet (not your office) to sip and reflect. The meditative time will soothe your frenzied brain, while the caffeine will give you just enough of a kick-start to get you through the rest of your day.

● **Clean your desk and clear out your email inbox.** Both are relatively mindless tasks that don't require great amounts of concentration or clear thinking, and both will leave you feeling more energised because you'll have accomplished something visible as well as having reduced energy-sapping clutter.

A cup of afternoon tea hits the spot.

● **Make an 'I was thinking of you' phone call.** To your wife, child, siblings, parents, a friend or a retired colleague. A 5 minute keep-in-touch call will lift your spirits for hours and reinvigorate you to get your work done.

● **Have an afternoon snack designed to get the blood flowing.** That doesn't mean a whole milk chocolate bar. The high glycaemic index in the chocolate bar (a measure of how high it pushes up your blood sugar) might give you a temporary boost, but once that jolt of sugar is gone, you'll sink faster than the stock market after an interest-rate hike. Instead, you want a snack that combines protein, fibre and complex carbohydrates (such as whole-grain crackers or raw vegetables) to raise your blood sugar levels steadily and keep them up. So opt for snacks such as:
● Low-fat milk and high-fibre cereal. Milk provides the protein as well as valuable fluid (tiredness is an early sign of dehydration), while the high-fibre cereal will curtail any sudden blood sugar rushes.
● Peanut butter spread on wholemeal crackers. Again, there's a good source of protein in peanut butter, a bit of fat for staying power (healthy fat, as well), coupled with the fibre and complex carbohydrates in the wholemeal crackers.
● Cut-up vegetables dipped into hummous. These days, you can buy both these ingredients at just about any food shop. Eaten together, you get the high fibre, antioxidants and valuable vitamins of the vegetables, coupled with the fibre and protein of the hummous.
● Tomato or vegetable juice with a handful of unsalted nuts. The nuts provide a healthy dose of protein and monounsaturated fat, while the tomato juice provides not only the lycopene and other phytonutrients found in tomatoes, but energy-sustaining liquid as well.

● A piece of Edam or low-fat cheese and an apple. Portable, easy and a great pair. The cheese, with its fat and protein, cushions the fruit sugars from the apple, while the apple provides you with one all-important fruit serving for the day, along with a healthy dollop of antioxidants and fibre (be sure to eat the skin).

☆ **Go for a 10 minute walk and resist that chocolate bar.** When American researchers compared study participants who ate a chocolate bar or who walked briskly for 10 minutes, they found the chocolate bar subjects felt more tense in the hour afterwards, while those who walked not only had higher energy levels for 1 to 2 hours afterwards, but also reduced their tension.

● **Defer the work you most want to do to the time of day when you least feel like working.** Get through the routine work in the early morning so it's done, then stave off the midday doldrums with a task you really enjoy.

● **Drink a cup of caffeinated coffee or tea.** The caffeine will perk you up; studies also find it will enhance your memory and make you more productive on tasks requiring concentration.

● **Put a drop of peppermint oil in your hand and briskly rub** your hands together, then rub them over your face (avoid your eyes). Peppermint is a known energy-enhancing scent.

● **Roll your shoulders forwards, then backwards,** timing each roll with a deep breath in and out. Repeat for 2 minutes.

● **Consider a morsel of dark chocolate.** This is not a licence to overindulge, but dark chocolate does have some unique

A small piece of dark chocolate is a healthy treat.

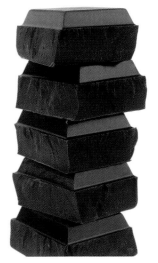

advantages. Unlike milk chocolate, it is truly a healthy food, closer to the category of nuts than sweets, given the high levels of healthy fat and antioxidants it contains. Plus, it has abundant fibre and magnesium. Additionally, it provides a little caffeine, as well as a satisfyingly decadent feeling. But don't eat more than one square.

Chew some 'spicy' gum. Chewing gums with strong minty flavours are stimulating, and the mere act of chewing is something of a tonic to a brain succumbing to lethargy. Plus, chewing stimulates saliva, which helps to clear out bacteria responsible for cavities and gum disease from lunch. Just be sure to choose sugar-free gum.

● **Plan group activities for midday.** If you often work on your own, try to organise work involving others at the time of day when your concentration might otherwise be waning. We are social animals, and interactions always rev us up. But make sure it's an interesting, interactive activity. Sitting in a room listening to someone else drone on and on will just send you snoozing.

● **Do your filing.** It's a physical activity that gets you up from your desk, bending and pulling and stretching. Plus, you can lose yourself in it, and any activity that enables you to get into a 'flow' will help to pull you through the doldrums.

● **Take 10 minutes for isometric exercises.** Isometric exercises involve nothing more than tensing a muscle and holding it. For instance, with your arm held out, tense your biceps and triceps at the same time and hold for 5 to 10 seconds. You can do this with your calf muscles, thigh muscles (front and back), chest,

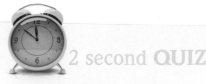

2 second QUIZ

Coffee or tea?
ANSWER: **TEA.**
Choose black or green tea. These are jammed with heart-healthy antioxidants that provide more than just an energy-boosting punch; as well as contributing to healthier arteries, they may also help to prevent cancer.

abdomen, buttocks, shoulders and back. If you wanted to, you could work a rotation, or cycle, of isometric exercises involving almost your entire body into your desk job every day. The total workout would be quite significant, despite never interrupting your work or causing you to break into a sweat. Plus, you're not only toning your body, you're toning your mind.

All day long...

● **Weave variety into your working day.** Tedium taxes the mind and induces somnolence. Most studies suggest that concentration on anything wanes after an hour, and is pretty near to pitiful at 90 minutes. So divide your tasks to maximise a balance between variety and productivity. For instance, if you have a large report you need to get out, work on it for 30 minutes, switch to something else for 30 minutes, then return to it.

● **Keep a rosemary plant in your office.** Not only will sharing your space with a live, growing thing provide its own mood boost, but studies find the scent of rosemary to be energising. Whenever you need a boost, just rub a sprig between your fingers to release the fragrance into the air. Or, if you're really wiped out, rub a sprig on your hands, face and neck.

At the **GYM**

If you are one of the minority of people who regularly go to a gym for exercise, then congratulations! It means you have the right priorities and terrific discipline. But it's fair to say that at times, even for committed exercisers, motivation often flags, and there are days when it requires a Herculean effort just to put on your workout clothes and walk through the gym doors.

If you're lucky, the sights and sounds of exercise are all you need to motivate you to get moving. At other times, you still may not have the slightest urge to get started. For those days, this chapter is for you. Here are the easy ways to get the most out of your workout.

16 IDEAS FOR HEALTHIER, EASIER WORKOUTS

☆ **Avoid the mirrors.** Many fitness centres line exercise rooms with mirrors to allow you to watch your form as you work out. Yet a study of 58 women found that those who exercised in front of a mirror felt less calm and more fatigued after 30 minutes of working out than those who exercised without staring at their reflections. One exercise chain, Curves, deliberately designs its small gyms without mirrors so that women can concentrate on each other and the workout rather than on how they look. Other gyms are beginning to offer 'reflection-free' zones. If yours doesn't, mention the idea – and the study – to the gym manager.

👟 **Try using aromatherapy oils known to enhance energy,** such as rosemary. Mix them with water and store them in a squirt bottle in your gym bag. Give your gym clothing a few squirts before leaving the dressing room so you can smell the oil as you work out. If you're in the midst of a more meditative, slower-paced workout, such as Pilates or yoga, try lavender oil instead of rosemary.

👟 **Create your own personal gym-mix tapes,** CDs or digital recordings, and listen to them as you work out. Researchers have found that people who listen to up-tempo music get significantly more out of their stationary bike workouts. They pedalled faster, produced more power and their hearts beat faster than when they listened to slow-tempo music or sounds with no tempo. Overall, they worked between 5 and 15 per cent harder while listening to the energising beat. Although the type of music you choose is up to you, pick something with a fast beat that makes you want to start dancing. You can custom-design your own exercise music to burn to a CD or download to an MP3 player.

Pick your
VIDEO OR DVD wisely

In a study completed at McMaster University in Ontario, Canada, exercise videos that featured super-skinny models with amazing muscles and revealing outfits made participants feel less confident about their fitness and less inclined to exercise in the future. Videos featuring an ultra-slender host surrounded by plumper, more normal-looking women reduced motivation even more. The researchers' hypothesis: seeing a thin instructor surrounded by fleshier participants intensified the participants' awareness of the thinness of the instructor.

To choose a motivating exercise DVD or class, look for a teacher you can trust, who has a fitness background and who must exercise to look great. In other words, DVDs created by personal trainers and exercise physiologists, or classes taught by them, will be more likely to motivate you than those hosted by supermodels and actresses.

👟 **Think of someone who irritates you.** Then step on the treadmill, exercise bike or elliptical machine and sweat out your aggression as you work out. You might even imagine that you are running an imaginary race against this person. You'll get a better workout – and blast away anger and stress at the same time.

😊 **Drink a bottle of water or juice on your way to the gym.** If you're already dehydrated, you'll feel overly fatigued during your session. When you're dehydrated, you can't work as hard, you don't feel as good and your mental function is compromised. So you won't get as much out of your workout.

👟 **Think you can and you will.** So simple, yet so often ignored, positive thinking can help you to power your way through a workout. In one study, exercisers who thought positively were more likely to stay active than those

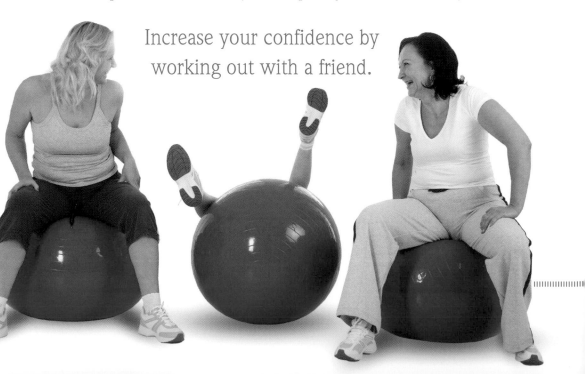

2 second QUIZ

Free weights vs. machines
ANSWER: **FREE WEIGHTS.**
With free weights, you can always work both sides of your body separately, eliminating muscle imbalances. Only some machines allow that. Not only that, you don't need a degree in astrophysics to figure out how to operate them or adjust them to your size and strength. Also, gym machines are generally designed for a male body. If you are short and slight, your body may be too small for the machine, no matter how much you adjust it. Finally, dumb-bells are inexpensive, small and nicely portable.

weren't watching TV than when they were. Although TV may take your mind off your workout, it also causes you to lose touch with your effort level. You unconsciously slow down or use poor form as you get caught up in what's on screen.

Work out with a friend. If you're feeling stale and are thinking of skipping your gym workouts, ask a friend to meet you for a gym date. As you walk or run on the treadmill, you can share stories of your day and encourage each other to work a bit harder. Your friend can also help you to find the courage to approach unfamiliar gym equipment, as it's easier to laugh off your foibles when you have a trusted companion nearby.

whose minds often uttered those two evil words, 'I can't.' Whenever you find yourself making excuses, replace any negative thoughts with positive messages such as, 'I feel great' or 'Bring it on.'

Turn off the TV when exercising. It's tempting to try to lose yourself in a TV programme as you slog away. But one study found that women worked out about 5 per cent harder when they

Wear the right shoes for the right class. Resist the urge to wear the old trainers you dug up from the back of the cupboard. Various fitness disciplines require specific types of footwear. The wrong shoes will not only make your workout feel harder, it could cause an injury. For example, wear running shoes for running, walking shoes for walking, and hard-bottomed cycling shoes for spinning (exercise on stationary bikes).

Increase your confidence by working out with a friend.

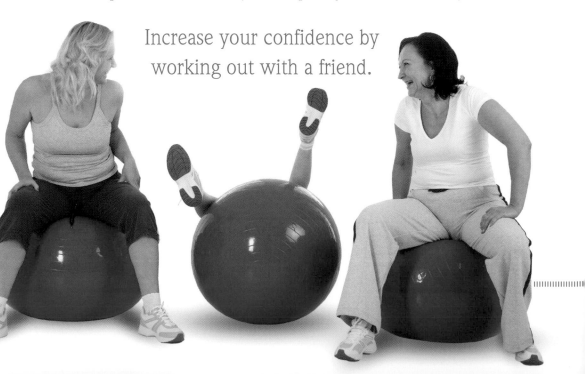

▶ Set a short-term workout goal. Of course, goals motivate you to work harder, and the best exercise programmes include measurable goals to achieve weeks or months down the road. Sometimes, though, when your motivation is drooping, a goal focusing on what you can complete over the next 30 minutes is what you need. So pick something achievable: maintain a sweat for 20 minutes, give your arms a good workout or cover 2 miles on the treadmill. A target like that gives you focus to get through.

Whenever you feel as if you're out of steam, hire a trainer. In just one session a trainer can open your eyes to a whole new world of workouts. (See 'What to look for in a trainer', opposite.)

Work out during the least crowded hours. You'll squeeze in a more effective workout in less time if you hit the gym during the slowest period of the day, often midafternoon. You won't have to wait in a queue for equipment or feel hassled in the changing room.

Change your routine every three to four weeks. This will keep your body guessing – improving your results – and fuel your motivation. In the weights room, alternate exercises and modify the way you lift weights. If you usually do two sets of 15 reps, complete one set of 15, then increase the weight for another set of 8 reps. On cardio equipment, switch from the treadmill to the stair stepper etc. Mix up your exercise classes as well, switching around from Pilates to aerobic dance to yoga to kickboxing.

☺ Slow down. In one American study, participants who lifted slowly – taking at least 14 seconds to complete one repetition – gained more strength than participants

What to look for **IN A TRAINER**

'Working out with a professional personal trainer/ fitness instructor not only focuses you on maintaining a consistent training programme, but also keeps your exercise routine exciting,' says Claire Small, director of physiotherapy at Pure Sports Medicine in London. 'A trainer can also show you the most effective exercises for your problem areas and help you to achieve the greatest results in the shortest amount of time.' To find the best trainer for you, follow these pointers:

● Choose a trainer with a degree in fitness, such as sports and exercise science, or exercise physiology.

● Make sure the trainer is on the Register of Exercise Professionals. In addition, he or she should also be a member of the UK Strength and Conditioning Association or the National Strength and Conditioning Association, which is US-based but recognised worldwide.

● Opt for a trainer you feel motivates you. Fire your trainer if he or she cancels or is always late.

who lifted at a rate of 7 seconds per rep. Slower lifting may help increase strength because it prevents you from using momentum or improper techniques.

Put your mind behind every move. Rather than daydreaming through your workouts, put as much mental emphasis on what you do at the gym as you do at work – or at least should do! For example, when doing a strength exercise, feel the muscle contract as you lift. This will help you to tune into your technique.

Invent a competition with the person on the next treadmill. If you're on the treadmill and you're bored, glance at the display on someone else's nearby treadmill. If you're walking at 3.5 miles per hour and he or she is chugging away at 4mph, see if you can increase your speed and catch up, as if it were a race. The other person won't even know you're racing.

Running ERRANDS

Like death and taxes, there's no escaping having to run errands.
Supermarket, chemist, dry-cleaner, library, post office. Pick up, drop off, wait for children – or parents. If you're not careful, you can spend more than half of your leisure time in your car seat running errands.

So what does any of that have to do with health? Plenty. All of those errands stress you out and suck you dry of energy. They also eat up hours that would be better spent exercising, relaxing, cooking, having fun – the healthy stuff of life. So the goal here is to get you through your errands faster, easier and with less stress. Just be sure to use the time you gain wisely.

19 WAYS TO GET THINGS DONE QUICKER WHILE HAVING MORE FUN

Group your errands. This is a golden rule: never run a single errand at a time. You'll save time, petrol, energy and stress hormones by grouping your errands into batches. If you have to drop a child at a piano lesson, you can also go via the bank and deposit a cheque, pop into the supermarket for milk and bread or pick up the dry-cleaning.

Run your errands at quiet times. In other words, not at the weekend (when the vast majority of people run their errands). Instead, make sure your dry-cleaner, bank, doctor, supermarket, etc., are near work so you can take care of these mundane tasks on your way into or out of work, or during your lunch hour. You'll avoid the packed shops and heavy traffic at the weekends, and have those two days just for you and your family. One of the best times to grocery shop? After dinner, when the children are in bed. One parent stays at home and one goes to the supermarket. You'll be in and out in half the time it takes with children in tow.

● **Create an errand centre in your house.** This is where library books that need to be returned, the dry-cleaning that needs to be dropped off, or the packages that need to be posted, all live. Everything in one place (ideally near the door you use most often) will make it easier to run 'bulk' errands. Another option: keep these things in your car, in the passenger seat. They'll be a visual reminder of all you need to do.

● **Keep an errand list with you at all times.** This includes both the ordinary errands that must be done (dry-cleaning, library, post office), but also those little things you keep forgetting (pick up socks for the six year old, make vet appointment for the dog, buy underwear for partner, find organic potting compost). Use a sturdy notebook that you carry with you at all times, and make sure the rest of your family knows where it is so they can add things to the list.

● **Buy in bulk.** The less often you have to go shopping for mundane items such as toilet paper, paper towels, dog food, cat litter, toothpaste, deodorant, tampons, etc., the less time you'll spend running errands. Storage space tight? Most of these items will fit under the bed quite nicely.

● **Always include a little fun.** List all the things you find joyful. Maybe it's reading a novel, writing in your diary or hitting a few golf balls on a spring afternoon. Now, plan to include one of these items in any extended errand run. Take a novel with you as you head to the post office; you can read it in the queue. Carry your diary in your glove compartment – jot down a few lines as you're waiting for the car to be washed. Or ride your bike to the shops, then take a spin around a local park or nearby countryside.

● **Turn waiting time into you time.** Any time you're stuck in a queue, shift the negative, glass-half-empty thinking ('I don't have time for this') into positive, glass-half-full thinking ('Ahhh! A few minutes of peace'). Close your eyes (yes, while you're standing there in the queue) and picture yourself in the most peaceful place you can imagine. It could be a desert at sunrise, the vast ocean (and you in a lone canoe) or the middle of a massage in a luxurious spa. Let your mind go and take several long, deep breaths. Now how do you feel?

Buy in bulk and you'll save precious time.

Use the internet for as many errands as possible. These days, you can bank online, order office supplies, buy garden perennials, shop for shoes and do your grocery shopping online. The internet, used sensibly, can save you hours of time and immeasurable stress. Worried about giving a credit card number over the internet? If the website uses a secured server, then it is safer than giving your credit card over the phone and, in some cases, using it at a shop.

● **Keep an 'errand bag' in the car at all times.** This includes such things as bills that need to be paid, stationery and envelopes for writing letters (yes, letters!), a variety of greetings cards (birthdays, thank you, 'just thinking of you'), pens, an envelope of coupons, your calendar, magazines that you haven't read and a good book. Then whenever you're sitting in a waiting room, stuck in traffic, waiting for a child's over-long football practice to end, you can also be completing other tasks on your list and/or catching up on your reading.

● **Keep a cooler and a basket in your boot.** The cooler is to keep frozen and cold foods cold while you run errands; the basket is so you can carry parcels into the house without making umpteen trips.

● **Learn to run errands with your kids and not go crazy.** There are few things more stressful than being stuck in traffic with ice cream melting in the boot and a two year old melting down in the back seat. But today you're more likely than ever to be running your errands with children in tow. To cope:
● Run your errands at the right time of day for the child. If you've got a toddler, that's morning, before naptime.

Your children aren't the only ones who need a little motivation ... buy yourself some flowers.

● **Offer to run errands for an elderly neighbour or a mother with young children.** Studies find that helping others actually reduces our own stress hormones and makes us feel better.

☆ **Keep your grocery list on the computer.** Most weeks, you're buying the same things anyway; having a master list on your computer makes it easy to add and subtract items. Organise the list in the same order as the shop you usually use. So, for instance, if the produce section is the first area you see, fruit and vegetables should be first on your list. Hit the print button and off you go!

- Stock the car with snacks, juices and toys. Keep a cooler in the front with cold drinks and cut-up fruit that you can hand back to your toddler when he or she gets grumpy. Have stocks of toys that come out only when you're running errands.
- Keep an extra nappy bag in the car. This way, you don't have to worry about forgetting something. Make sure the bag is stocked with nappies, wipes, a change of clothes and nappy cream.
- Combine errands for you with a treat for your child. It could be lunch out, an ice cream or a trip to the park.
- Play games while you're shopping. Give a school-age child a calculator and ask him or her to add up the cost of the groceries as you go along. Let pre-school children put non-breakable items into the trolley. Toddlers can pick the colour of the tissues you buy, and will enjoy a game of peekaboo as you go round the aisles.
- Bring the right carrying equipment for babies and infants: a backpack type of carrier, or a front sling, both of which leave your hands free.
- Play a thinking game with older children to keep them disciplined and you relaxed. A good game is 'jotto'. You each pick a word with five letters, no two the same, and have to guess the other's word by stating five-letter words and being told how many letters match. Keeping track in your head is challenging, but fun.

● **Pay attention as you run your errands.** That is, rein in your racing mind and focus solely on the task at hand. Start by walking slowly and deliberately to and from your car to the shops. As you shop, focus on the colours and shapes of the produce and the rich scents from the bakery. Notice each step, each movement you make. By living mindfully in the moment – even while picking out Brussels sprouts – you are performing what relaxation experts call walking meditation. Do errands this way and you'll find yourself far more calm and engaged and, at the end, less exhausted and frustrated.

☺ **Buy yourself a treat.** Your children aren't the only ones who need a little motivation during errand running. So make sure you add one more item to your list – something nice for you. It could be flowers, a scented bath soap, an imported brand of beer or a fancy cheese.

● **Keep several bottles of water in the freezer.** When it's time to run errands in the summer, grab one of them to take with you. You'll have plenty of icy-cold water to drink as you go along.

● **Listen to inspirational tapes or books on CD** in the car while running errands. It's a lot more relaxing than the commercials, the DJs and the overall intensity of everyday radio.

● **Alternate tasks with your neighbours or children's friends.** For instance, one week you do the grocery shopping for your neighbour; the next week, she does it for you. Or she watches your children while you do the errands for both families (or vice versa). Another option: do errands with a friend. Not only will you benefit from the social support, but your children might just be better behaved if there's another adult there.

● **If you're a dad, run errands with your child.** An American study has found that children who clean, cook and do household errands with their fathers are better behaved and have more friends. An added bonus: the wives of these men find them more sexually attractive.

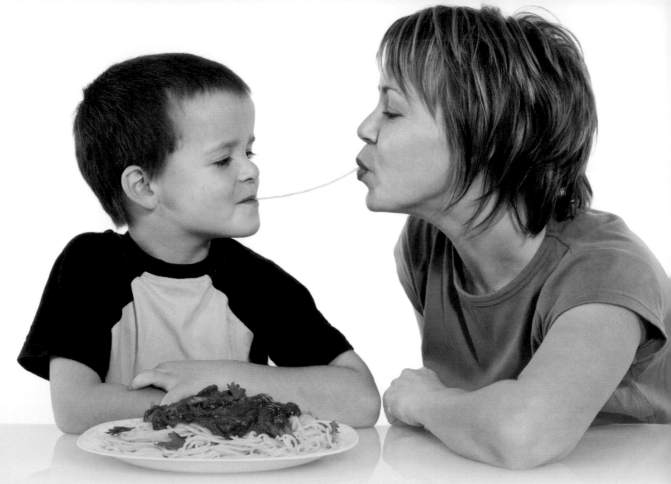

The **DINNER** routine

We're all busy. Whether it's working, caring for children, running errands, studying, volunteering or some combination of the above, we are all rushed off our feet. Too tired or unprepared to cook after 10 or 12 hours of perpetual busyness, we often take the easy path: a pizza or other takeaway food, a frozen meal. Yet such pre-prepared dishes are filled with salt, sugar and fat. Then there's the shortage of vegetables, fibre and vitamins, not to mention the portion sizes – often huge. There is a better way. Here are simple, realistic, easy tips to get you eating healthily at dinner again.

24 WAYS TO MAKE SUPPER SUPREMELY HEALTHY

☺ **Keep your kitchen tidy.** Families tend to congregate in the kitchen, bringing with them newspapers, post, schoolbags, schoolwork, toys and a thousand other little things. Don't allow it. Set a new policy: the kitchen is for cooking and, if you have room, eating only. Why? It's hard to get motivated about cooking if you have to clean up a mess first, not to mention what it does to your mood. The opposite also holds true: a clean, bright, inviting kitchen can be a wonderful oasis after a day of craziness.

☞ **Speaking of which, make your kitchen a place you like to be.** Is there music playing? Do you have a glass of wine? Is the evening sun shining through the window? Are the knives sharp, the vegetables fresh, the pots good quality, the worktops clutter-free? All of these contribute to your desire to make good food. If you don't enjoy being in your kitchen, do what you need to change that.

☆ **Plan a week's worth of dinners.** Many of us don't know what we're having for dinner as late as 4pm in the afternoon. Yet planning ahead takes just a few minutes. Here's how to do it. Every Friday night or Saturday morning, sit down with a pad of paper and your favourite cookbooks or some cookery magazines. Think about what's in your freezer and fridge, what your family likes to eat, what your upcoming week entails. Then plan out a week's worth of menus (you can always leave one night for takeaway pizzas). At the same time, write out your shopping list. Now stick the list of menus on the fridge or bulletin board so it's the first thing you see when you get home. Voilà! No more thinking ahead. If you need help or inspiration, consider an online meal planner, such as www.shoppingplanner.co.uk.

Healthy INVESTMENT

A panini machine
Panini are sandwiches grilled in a machine that looks like an oversized sandwich toaster and that presses all the ingredients together. Panini machines are widely available and turn an ordinary sandwich into a real treat. Keep whole-grain bread on hand at all times (bread freezes well). When you can't think of what to have for dinner, serving panini with various grilled veggies works beautifully.

☞ **Enjoy the cooking process.** Of course, not everyone loves cooking. But there's no reason to not like doing it. If the thought of cooking fills you full of dread, you need an attitude adjustment. Cooking is a pleasure, far easier than many non-cooks realise. For the sake of your health, your pleasure and your wallet, you should learn – or relearn – the pleasures of cooking. Make it a project. Spend time with your friends and family while they cook so that you can absorb the methods and routines. Consider taking a class, or buy an introductory cookbook. Most of all, lose your fear. It is harder to be a bad cook than a good cook, particularly if you use good ingredients.

☞ **Delegate, delegate, delegate.** If you have children aged ten-plus or another adult who gets home before you do, get them started on dinner. For example, you might ask your partner to pick up ingredients on the way home, your teen to start chopping vegetables for the salad and fill the pasta pot with water, and your pre-teen to gather necessary ingredients for a given recipe and put them on the worktop for you, preheat the oven and set the table. Yes, they may think of it as a chore, but if you build in a little opportunity for them to 'create' (for example, with place cards for dinner, more slowly than carbohydrates, keeping your appetite under control for a longer period of time.

☞ Turn off the television during dinner. A study has found that the more television and videos students watched, the fewer fruits and vegetables they ate. Researchers theorise that television programmes and commercials depict unhealthy foods, causing people to reach more often for soft drinks and crisps rather than fruit and vegetables. A separate study found that watching television during dinner reduced fruit and vegetable consumption during the meal.

▌▌▌▶ If your children won't eat what you put on their plate, bite your tongue. Hassling children over their eating habits during dinner actually causes children – and their parents – to eat less well, according to one study. Both the children and their parents consumed more fat during meals when they argued over eating behaviour. The stress from the argument may have led to cravings for fatty comfort foods rather than an appetite for Brussels sprouts and spinach.

☞ Instead of forcing kids to clean their plates, enforce a one-bite rule. Encourage your children to take one bite out of all the foods on their plate. If, after one bite, they still don't want to eat their spinach or broccoli, let them push it aside. This technique encourages children to try new foods, but doesn't create a stressful eating experience. Also, involve young children in preparing foods you want them to try. A sense of ownership makes them bolder.

☞ Avoid alcohol before your dinner. In a study conducted at the University of Liverpool, men who drank a glass of beer 30 minutes before a meal ate more during the meal than men who had a soft drink. They also ate more fatty, salty foods and felt hungrier after the meal than men who didn't drink. Alcohol stimulates the appetite, so if you don't want to eat too much, avoid alcohol or enjoy one glass with, not before, your meal.

☞ No ideas and need to lose a few pounds? Serve cereal. This handy standby provides plenty of vitamins and minerals, together with some protein from the milk, and fibre, if you choose a high-fibre cereal. More importantly, it could help the entire family to lose weight. In one study, people who ate a bowl of cereal instead of lunch or dinner consumed on average 640kcal less a day and lost an average of 4lb (just under 2kg) of fat in two weeks. Or make up a great big bowl of muesli for the whole family, mixing cut-up fruit with low-fat muesli cereal with or without nuts, fat-free plain yoghurt and honey.

☞ Have breakfast for dinner. A great 'breakfast' option for dinner is an omelette. It's quick and easy to make, a good protein source and relatively low in calories. Fill it with veggies instead of cheese, and you have a complete meal in a frying pan.

☞ Use parts of last night's dinner for tonight's meal. This allows you to cook once and eat twice. For example, if you have roast chicken one night, use the leftovers to serve up chicken fajitas or chicken salad the next. Prepare all key protein foods – chicken, turkey, fish, etc. – in larger-than-needed amounts so they will last two nights instead of one. Do the same with rice and other grain-based side dishes. Serve as a side dish one night and use the leftovers to make a casserole, stir-fry or soup the next.

The **AFTER-DINNER** routine

Dinner is finished, the dishes are done and you're looking at a lovely 3 hours ahead of you before your body begins sending go-to-sleep signals. You could sit in front of the TV, as so many people do these days. Or you could choose to do one of the following and sneak a little health into your evening. This section starts off with pleasure-based ideas, then shifts into more practical ways to spend your evening time.

24 IDEAS FOR HEALTHIER, MORE PLEASURABLE EVENINGS

☺ **Go for an after-dinner walk.** What better time for a hand-in-hand stroll through the neighbourhood? To make it interesting, play a game of learning two new things about your neighbours on each walk, either through observation or conversation. It could be that the Smiths have painted their living room red (something you spot through the window), or that Mrs Walker has a new car. Playing this kind of game on your walk will make it go quicker and keep it more interesting. The best bonus: the health-promoting effects of the walk.

● **Play a game with your partner or children.** Try a board game, work on a puzzle or opt for a rousing game of cards. Not only will it keep the television off, but it will make those brain cells work a lot harder. And the social bonding with your loved ones contributes mightily to emotional and physical health. Stumped for choices? Go back in time to when you were a teenager – try games such as backgammon, dominoes, draughts or chess. Crossword puzzles are great fun, as

are visual, number and logic puzzles. Do you have a dartboard, pool table or table-tennis table? Wear them out.

● **Go up to your partner, put your arms round his/her waist,** and begin kissing the back of his/her neck. Hopefully, this will lead to something more. In addition to the obvious benefits of sex, you'll also be raising your heart rate, sending immune-boosting endorphins to your brain and extending your life. One study found that sexually active men lived longer than those who made love less often. The study covered men, but it is likely to apply to women too.

● **Do something totally mindless for 30 minutes.** It could be watching the most mind-numbing programme you can find on TV, holding a computer solitaire tournament with yourself, soaking in a steamy, scented bath or just lying on the couch listening to a favourite piece of music and staring at the ceiling. The idea

Lose yourself in a good book.

here is that your mind is disengaged; it is not focused on anything, but is allowed to run free in a kind of 'active meditation'.

⭐ **Slowly sip a glass of really good wine once in a while.** The definition of 'really good wine' depends on your tastes. If you're used to bog-standard boxed wine, then a £10 bottle of merlot is just the ticket. If you're a moderate oenophile, you might reach for a £25 bottle of Bordeaux. The idea is that you savour this one glass. While you're identifying the flavours and the elements in the bouquet, the wine, if it's red, will be providing significant heart-healthy antioxidants, shown to reduce your risk of heart disease.

● **Get lost in a book.** Or a magazine or a newspaper. Rekindle your love of reading. It's so much more rewarding for you than watching television. And it's much healthier, because it keeps your brain highly active and engaged.

⭐ **Savour a piece of dark gourmet chocolate.** Gram for gram, chocolate contains more healthy antioxidants, which repair damage to cells and prevent cholesterol from oxidising (making it stickier), than any of the other antioxidant champions, including tea, blueberries and grape juice. Plus, it's well known for its ability to soothe a troubled mind. It takes only one piece to provide the perfect post-dinner sweetness we often crave. Keep the chocolate dark – it has the most antioxidants – and plain. You don't need the extra sugar and calories from caramel and other goodies.

● **On a dark, clear night, go outside and lie down in your back garden** and stare at the stars. Feel the immensity of the world as you view the heavens. Think about any problems you've been wrestling with and put them into context with the trillions of stars that are up there. If you find you enjoy this, consider learning about the stars with a star atlas. Or take a walk when the moon is full. The magic and mysticism of a moonlit night will energise you and provide an unexpected burst of positive thinking.

● **Go to sleep at 8pm.** Many of us are sleep-deprived. So every now and again, pretend you're six years old, put on flannel pyjamas, get into bed at 8pm and turn out the light.

● **Give yourself a pedicure.** Fill a basin with warm water and a few drops of peppermint oil. Soak your feet in it until the water cools, then pumice away the rough skin on your soles. Massage a scented lotion all over your feet, inhaling the lovely scent and feeling your skin soften with every stroke. Trim your toenails, push back your cuticles and, if you desire, polish your toenails in a colour you'd never dare wear on your fingernails. If you can, convince your partner to give you a foot massage.

● **Ask your partner, or even an older child or a friend, to wash your hair.** Having your hair washed and your scalp massaged is an unexpected luxury that will help wash away the stress of the day.

● **Put a CD (whatever music you like dancing to)** on the stereo and dance for 20 minutes. Jazz and cheek-to-cheek dancing not your thing? Fine, slip some high-energy rock music into the CD and pretend you're in a mosh pit. Either way, you'll get 20 minutes of physical activity and, if you're doing the mosh pit thing, you'll burn as many calories as if you were jogging. An added bonus: improved coordination and, if you do a lot of dips, some good stretches. Plus, this is a great way for younger parents to engage their kids in physical activity – the whole family can let themselves go, dancing energetically until just one is left standing.

☺ **Make a yoghurt smoothie for dessert.** Toss a frozen banana, a pot of plain or vanilla yoghurt, a handful of blueberries and a teaspoon of honey into the blender along with some crushed ice. Blend the mixture until it is thick and smooth. The combination of the antioxidants in the blueberries, the potassium in the banana and the live bacteria in the yoghurt will give you a health boost that no vitamin can match. Specific conditions you have just helped to protect yourself against: urinary tract infection (blueberries), high blood pressure (banana) and yeast infection or irritable bowel syndrome (yoghurt).

● **Sip a cup of camomile or mint tea.** The camomile will help you to sleep and the mint will aid your digestion.

● **Set a timer and write your diary for 10 minutes.** Many people don't want to keep a diary because they can't stand the sense of responsibility it brings to write in it every night. But if you know you have

Interact with your pet and your stress will melt away.

only 10 minutes, suddenly what seemed like a chore takes less time than washing the dishes. Not sure what to write? Just try listing what you did that day. Write down five things that made you smile. List five things that made you angry – and why. Numerous studies attest to the stress-busting power of regular diary writing. Plus, it's fun to leaf back through your diary and see what you were doing a year before.

● **Express yourself.** Go one better than a diary: compose a letter to a friend, write some emails or a missive to your MP or local councillor, or write a short story. Writing is wonderful brain activity, and who doesn't benefit from learning how to express themselves better?

● **Write down your entire to-do list for the next day.** It takes 5 minutes, yet the peace of mind it brings is priceless. Instead of running a to-do list over and over in your mind – making your responsibilities morph into gargantuan proportions – you can enjoy the rest of your evening and have a better shot at sleeping.

● **Play with your dog or cat for 15 minutes.** Studies show significant stress-reduction benefits from pets, particularly those that, like dogs and cats, can interact with you. Looking for ideas? Find an old sock and get your dog to try to pull it out of your hand. Teach your cat to 'fetch' by tossing a crumpled piece of paper. Hide treats around the house and watch your dog or cat go on a treasure hunt. Don't have a pet? Get one!

▐▐▐▶ **Pack your (or your children's) lunch for tomorrow,** and also lay out your clothes, check your briefcase and make sure the children's school stuff is by the front door. The health benefits are clear: this will avoid the surge in stress hormones the following morning that comes from rushing around like a stockbroker on Black Monday while screaming at the children, ripping your tights and spilling juice on your silk shirt.

😊 **Once a week, hold a 'chore-free' night.** Order pizza and eat on paper plates, leave dishes unwashed, forget the laundry, don't even wipe the worktops. Arrange lifts for the children to football practice or piano. This is your night to be as lazy (or productive in other ways) as you like. Maybe you have a hobby that you never seem to have the time to get to. This is your night for you. Don't let anything – especially your guilt – get in the way. If your life is too hectic to pull it off once a week, make it every other week or once a month. But make it some time.

⬤ **Have a cooking fest.** Tonight, cook meals for the next two weeks to stock up your freezer. Try easy-to-double recipes such as lasagne or meatballs (use turkey to reduce the heart-clogging saturated fat) or lentil or aubergine casserole.

⬤ **Change into nightclothes and slippers early in the evening.** Even before dinner. It will help separate the 'daytime you' from the 'evening you', and be a constant reminder throughout the evening to relax.

Healthy INVESTMENT

A diary
Don't think of diaries as a private place for teenage girls to write about their newest crushes. Every single adult – be it man or woman – can benefit from having a good-quality notebook to record observations, thoughts, opinions and reminders. At the front or the back of the diary, set aside pages for lists of books to read, music to buy, restaurants to try, even friends to call. While shopping for a diary, buy a nice pen to go with it. Keep them by your bedside so they're always ready for you at bedtime (and in the morning, when dreams and ideas are fresh). Don't feel compelled to write every night, but remember: the more you write, the more you'll want to write in the future. You'll probably find that a private diary is an outstanding way to diffuse stress, clear your mind and organise your thoughts.

😊 **Clean out one cupboard in your house.** This chore takes no more than 30 minutes, and leaves you with a sense of accomplishment, yet without any added stress because the task is simple and unchallenging, yet satisfying.

⬤ **Do your weekend shopping and chores.** Why buy your groceries or go clothes shopping when everyone else is doing it? Make Saturday a fun day, not an errand and shopping day. The shops are much emptier and shopping is less stressful on weekday evenings.

Reminder

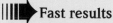 **Fast results**
These are tips that deliver benefits particularly quickly – in some cases, immediately.

😊 **Easy gains**
These are health boosters that offer the best value for the least amount of effort.

☆ **Super-effective**
This is advice that scientific research or widespread usage by experts has shown to be especially effective.

The CLEANING routine

You may not realise it, but your house is hazardous to your health. Insect droppings, dust mites, bacteria-laden sponges, spoiled food – all can contribute to a plethora of health problems ranging from allergies and asthma to gastrointestinal upsets. In fact, an American germ guru, Dr Charles P. Gerba, professor of microbiology at the University of Arizona, says you're more likely to get sick at home than nearly anywhere else in your life (except maybe hospitals). What's scarier is that the cure for a dirty home can be worse than the problem as we attack germs with more and more toxic chemicals. Many cleaning products contain volatile organic compounds (VOCs), which can cause eye, nose and lung irritation, as well as rashes, headaches, nausea, asthma and, in some cases, cancer. There is a solution. Here's what the leading 'green' cleaners recommend.

12 TIPS FOR HEALTH-FRIENDLY CLEANING

● **Clean in an organised manner.** There's no point in mopping the floor only to dust the ceiling fan next and deposit a grey film over everything again. To clean well – and that means to clean healthily – you need to clean efficiently, avoiding going back and forth around a room. Instead, work using a systematic approach. Think in terms of left to right, top to bottom. Begin with ceilings and walls, and work your way down to windows and furniture, finishing with the floors.

☆ **Clean the things you'd never think to clean.** For instance, your mattress is a magnet for allergy-causing dust mites. Washing the mattress cover in very hot water (60°C or more) every month, and wiping down the top of the mattress with hot water, can go a long way towards reducing morning stuffiness. Other areas often ignored:
● Indoor rubbish bins. Particularly those in the kitchen and bathroom. Emptying them isn't the same as cleaning them. Scrub them regularly to make sure germs aren't germinating.
● Shower curtains. They get wet most days, and they often stay wet, making them a perfect home for mould.
● Automatic dishwashers. Take a close look at the edges of the door on your dishwasher. Many are breeding grounds for mould and mildew. The same is true of the rubber cushioning that surrounds some fridge doors.
● The fireplace. A clogged chimney is not only unhealthy, it can kill you if it ignites or, in the case of a gas fireplace, becomes blocked, sending dangerous carbon monoxide fumes into the house.
● HVAC filters. These filters are designed to filter out allergy-causing dust from the air, but if they're clogged, they're more harmful than helpful.

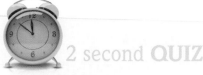
● **Dust with worn-out wool socks or a corner of an old wool blanket** or jumper. Wool creates static when rubbed on a surface. One wipe can keep your furniture dust-free without polish or spray.

● **Polish silver with toothpaste.** Some silver polishes contain petroleum distillates, ammonia or other hazardous ingredients. Instead, dab on toothpaste with your finger or rub it on with a cloth. Rinse with warm water and polish with a soft cloth. For larger trays and bowls, use a paste made of bicarbonate of soda mixed with water on a wet sponge.

☆ **Clean your drains the non-toxic way.** Chemical drain cleaners (also called drain openers) are extremely corrosive and dangerous, containing such toxic ingredients as lye or sulphuric acid. Even the vapours are harmful. Instead, pour a pot of boiling water or toss a handful of bicarbonate followed by 125ml of vinegar down the drain weekly. Also effective, particularly in preventing blockages, are many brands of enzymatic cleaners found in pet shops.

The **SLEEP** routine

Blessed sleep – the holy grail of health. Did you know that some researchers believe a chronic lack of sleep may lead to insulin resistance, a risk factor for diabetes? That's just for starters. Sleep deprivation can also alter your levels of thyroid and stress hormones, potentially affecting everything from your memory to your immune system, heart and metabolism. Of course, lack of sleep can kill you instantly. According to Jim Horne of the Sleep Research Laboratory at Loughborough University, an estimated 10 per cent of all road traffic accidents, and 20 per cent of all motorway accidents, are sleep-related. Yet only one in ten of us says we always sleep well and an estimated 20 per cent of people worldwide experience insomnia. A good night's sleep is one of the best things for your health, so pick three of these tips to follow each night until you get all that you need.

20 WAYS TO ACHIEVE A DEEP, UNINTERRUPTED SLEEP

☺ **Create a transition routine.** This is something you do every night before bed. It could be as simple as letting the cat out, turning out the lights, turning down the heat, washing your face and brushing your teeth. Or it could be a series of yoga or meditation exercises. Regardless, it should be consistent. As you begin to move into your 'nightly routine', your mind will get the signal that it's time to chill out, physiologically preparing you for sleep.

ᶻᶻ **Figure out your body cycle.** Do you ever find that you get really sleepy at 10pm, that the sleepiness passes, and that by the time the late news comes on, you're wide awake? Some experts believe sleepiness comes in cycles. Push past a period of tiredness and you probably won't be able to fall asleep very easily for a while. If you've noticed these kinds of rhythms in your own body clock, use them to your advantage. When sleepiness comes, get to bed. Otherwise, it might be a long time until you're ready for sleep again.

ᶻᶻ **Sprinkle just-washed sheets and pillowcases with lavender water** and iron them before making up your bed. The scent is scientifically proven to promote relaxation, and the repetition and mindlessness of ironing will soothe you. Or put lavender water in a perfume atomiser and spray above your bed just before climbing in.

ᶻᶻ **Hide your clock under your bed** or on the bottom shelf of your bedside cabinet, where its glow won't disturb you. That way, if you do wake up in the middle of the night or have problems sleeping, you won't fret over how late it is and how much sleep you're missing.

ᶻᶻ **Change your pillow.** If you're constantly pounding it, turning it over and upside down, the poor pillow deserves a break. Find a fresh new pillow from the linen cupboard, put a sweet-smelling case on it and try again.

ᶻᶻ **Pyjamas or naked?** The answer is pyjamas. Warm skin helps to slow down your blood's circulation, cooling your internal temperature and generally contributing to a deeper sleep. Just don't overdo it. Your body goes through a few cool–warm cycles as the night passes, so you want pyjamas, sheets and covers that keep you comfortable through these changes.

ᶻᶻ **Tidy your bedroom and paint it a soothing sage green.** Or some other soothing colour. First, remove the clutter from your bedroom – it provides a distraction and stands in the way of a good night's sleep. A soothing colour provides a visual reminder of sleep, relaxing you as you lie in bed reading or preparing for sleep.

ᶻᶻ **Choose the right pillow.** One Swedish study found that neck pillows, which resemble a rectangle with a depression in the middle, can actually enhance the quality of your sleep as well as reduce neck pain. The ideal neck pillow should be soft and not too high, provide neck support and be allergy tested and washable, researchers found. A pillow with two supporting cores received the best rating from the 55 people who participated in the study. Another study found that water-filled pillows

Sage green walls make a soothing bedroom.

provided the best night's sleep when compared to participants' usual pillows or a roll pillow, and yet another study rated 'cool' pillows best, so choose one made of natural fibres, which release heat better and keep your head cooler than polyester. If you're subject to allergies or find you're often stuffed up when you awake in the morning, try a hypoallergenic pillow.

ᶻᶻᴢ **Switch to heavier curtains over the windows** if you find it difficult to drop off. Even the light from streetlights, a full moon or your neighbour's house can interfere with the circadian rhythm changes you need to fall asleep.

Healthy **INVESTMENT**

A good mattress
A survey of 400 people found that 8 in 10 thought a bad mattress could cause sleep problems. Ironically, nearly half said they had a 'bad' or 'very bad' mattress. First off, you need a new mattress if yours is ten years old or even older. Also consider how lumpy it is – ditch your mattress if its topography resembles a mountain range, with its peaks, valleys and slopes. Another warning sign is waking up feeling sore or stiff, despite not being physically active the day before. Although no one mattress works best for everybody, there are some guidelines to follow:
● **Size.** Make sure you buy one that's larger than you think you will need, especially if you sleep with someone else.
● **Firmness.** This is strictly an individual decision. But make sure you try out any mattress in the shop. Lie on it. Roll over. Get into your typical sleeping position.
● **Frame.** Make sure you get a sturdy, good-quality frame, one with at least ten slats and a fifth leg as a centre support.
● **Maintenance.** Turn your mattress over and upside down at least every three months.

ᶻᶻᴢ **Move your bed away from any outside walls.** This will help to cut down on noise, which a Spanish study found could be a significant factor in insomnia. If the noise is still bothering you, try a white-noise machine, or just turn on a fan.

ᶻᶻᴢ **Tuck a hot-water bottle between your feet** or wear a pair of ski socks to bed in winter. The science is a little complicated, but warm feet help your body's internal temperature get to the optimal level for sleep. Essentially, you sleep best when your core temperature drops. By warming your feet, you make sure blood flows well through your legs, allowing your trunk to cool.

ᶻᶻᴢ **Kick your dog or cat out of your bedroom.** A 2002 research study found that one in five pet owners sleep with their pets. The study also found that dogs and cats created one of the biggest impediments to a good night's sleep since the discovery of caffeine. One reason? The study found that 21 per cent of the dogs and 7 per cent of the cats snored!

ᶻᶻᴢ **Sleep alone.** One of the greatest disruptors of sleep is your loved one dreaming away next to you. He might snore, she might kick or cry out. In fact, one study found that 86 per cent of women surveyed said their husbands snored, and half had their sleep interrupted by it. Men have it a bit easier: 57 per cent said their wives snored, while just 15 per cent found their sleep bothered by it. If you won't kick your partner out (or head to the guest room yourself), consider these anti-snoring tips:
● Get him (or her) to stop smoking. Cigarette smoking contributes to snoring.
● Feed him (or her) a light meal for dinner and avoid any alcohol, which can add to the snoring.

- Buy some earplugs and use them.
- Play soft music to drown out the noise.
- Present your lover with a gift-wrapped box of Breathe Right strips, which work by pulling the nostrils open wider. A Swedish study found they significantly reduced snoring.
- Make an appointment for your partner at a sleep centre. If nothing you do improves his or her snoring, your bedmate might be a candidate for a sleep test called polysomnography to see if sleep apnoea is the cause.

ᶻᶻZ **Munch a banana before bed.** It's a great natural source of melatonin, the sleep hormone, as well as tryptophan. The time-honoured tradition, of course, is warm milk, also a good source of tryptophan.

ᶻᶻZ **Take antacids straight after dinner, not before bed.** If you take antacids, take them after dinner – they contain aluminium, which appears to interfere with sleep.

ᶻᶻZ **Listen to a book on tape while you fall asleep.** Just as a bedtime story soothes and relaxes children, a calming book on tape (try poetry or a biography, but stay away from horror novels) can have the same effect with us grown-ups.

ᶻᶻZ **Simmer three to four large lettuce leaves in a cup of water** for 15 minutes. Remove from the heat, add two sprigs of mint, and sip just before you go to bed. Lettuce contains a sleep-inducing substance called lactucarium, which affects the brain in a similar way to opium (but without the risk of addiction)!

ᶻᶻZ **Use eucalyptus for a muscle rub.** The strongly scented herb provides a soothing feeling and relaxing scent.

Do **THREE** things...

If you can do only three things, try these to get a good night's sleep:

1 Allow one hour before bedtime for a relaxing activity. Watching the news or answering emails does not count. Better choices are reading or listening to soft music. As for sex … some people say it just wakes them up. So factor this into the timing of your bedtime routine.

2 If your mind is relaxed but your body is tense, do some low-intensity stretches and exercises to relax your muscles, especially those in your upper body, neck and shoulders. Before you go to bed, use light weights (1-2kg /3-5lb for women; 2-4kg/5-10lb for men) to exercise these muscles calmly. Do one set of eight to ten repetitions of a basic exercise for each upper body muscle.

3 Allow at least 3 hours between dinner and bedtime. The brain does not sleep well on a full stomach. If you know that you'll be busy the following day, have your big meal at lunchtime and a lighter meal as early as possible in the evening.

☆ **Take a hot bath 90 to 120 minutes before bedtime.** A study published in the journal *Sleep* found that women with insomnia who took a hot bath at this point (with the water temperature at approximately 40°C), slept much better that night. The bath increased their core body temperature, which abruptly dropped once they got out of the bath, readying them for sleep.

ᶻᶻZ **Give yourself a massage.** Slowly move the tips of your fingers around your eyes in a slow, circular motion. After a minute, move down to your mouth, then to your neck and the back of your head. Continue down your body until you're ready to drop off to sleep. Another option: ask your partner for a massage and massage each other on alternate nights.

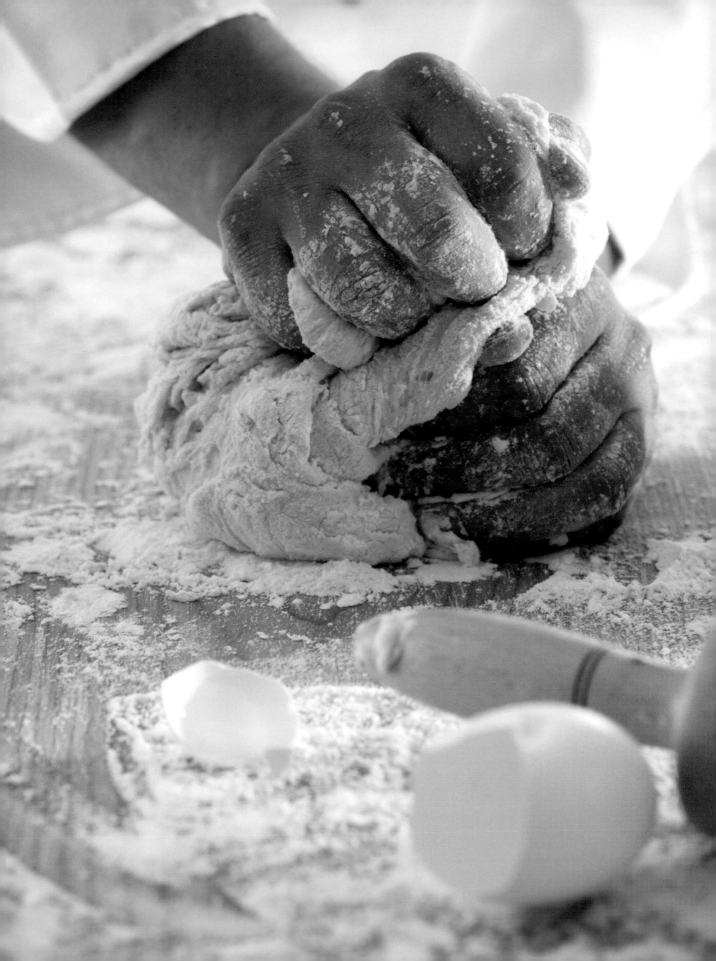

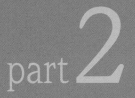

part 2

HEALTH BOOSTING COOKING

Probably the easiest and most effective way to improve your health is by adjusting your diet. Learn the best tricks for eating the right foods – and avoiding the bad.

FOOD shopping

The typical British man or woman does a main grocery shop roughly once a week, and almost a third of us do some top-up shopping too; the average family of four now spends well over £100 a week on food. So, why oh why does it often feel as if there's nothing to eat at home? Maybe you're not approaching the grocery shopping with the right attitude – or list. Follow the advice in this section to ensure you not only have well-stocked food cupboards for healthy eating, but are buying the right products at the right time in the right way. Learn what to look for on a product's nutrition label to ensure that you're getting the healthiest ingredients; see the panel on page 81 and for further research check out www.whatsinsideguide.com or www.eatwell.gov.uk.

25 TIPS FOR YOUR GROCERY LIST

Rule number one: buy fresh food! There is no simpler, no easier, nor plainer measure of the healthiness of your food than whether it comes to you in boxes and cans or is fresh from the farm or fields. If more than half of your shopping comprises pre-prepared foods, then you need to take your eating habits back to the healthy side by opting for more fresh vegetables, fruit, seafood, juices and dairy products.

Shop round the perimeter of the supermarket. That's where you'll find the fresh foods in many shops. If that's the case in your supermarket, avoid the central aisles and your shopping trip will be the healthier for it. Just dip into the aisles for the staples you know you need.

Think of the different sections (dairy, fresh produce, meat and so on) as separate shops within the supermarket. You wouldn't shop at every shop in the shopping centre, would you? Target only those that are safe to browse through – the fresh food sections, primarily – and steer clear of the danger areas (sweets, ice cream, crisps …).

Shop with a list. Organise your shopping list based on the tip above – that is, order it by the individual sections of the shop. This will get you out of the supermarket at the speed of light. If you're a woman, consider asking your husband or son to do the food shopping. US research shows that, compared to women, men are more likely to buy only what's on the list. But shopping with a list has benefits beyond speed and spending. By sticking rigidly to a well-planned shopping list, you can resist the seductive call of aisle upon aisle of junk food, thereby saving your family and yourself from an overload of empty calories.

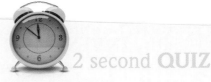

2 second QUIZ

Paper or plastic?
ANSWER: **PAPER.**

The debate over which bag is better for the environment is long and complicated. Yes, plastic can be recycled, but it's not as easy as recycling paper. And plastic production and processing require the use of toxic chemicals. Plus, plastic decomposes only when air and sunlight are present, whereas landfilled rubbish is buried. On the plus side, the newer bioplastics are made from renewable sources such as cornflour and vegetable oils, which are compostable. Meanwhile, although paper bags are made using manufacturing techniques that require water and air pollution, they are increasingly made from reprocessed materials and are more easily recycled and broken down. An even better bet: choose reusable cloth or string bags.

Food-shop on a full stomach. You've no doubt heard it before, but it's worth repeating. Walking through a supermarket with your tummy rumbling can make you vulnerable to buying anything that isn't moving. If you can't arrange to shop shortly after a meal, be sure to eat an apple and drink a large glass of water before heading into the shop.

Purchase a few days before food is fully ripe. There's no point in trying to buy fresh vegetables and fruit for your family if the bananas turn brown and the peaches go mushy two days after you get them home. Buy fruit that's still a day or two behind ripeness. It will still be hard to the touch; bananas will be green. Feel carefully for bruises on apples, check expiry dates on bagged produce and stay away from potatoes or onions that have started to sprout. If the fresh produce on the shelves looks a bit beyond its peak, including apparently healthy foods such as fruit juices, pre-made spaghetti sauces and even bread. If corn syrup is listed as one of the four main ingredients (usually near the top), for your good health's sake, avoid it.

✅ **Look for fibre.** You want at least 1 to 2g of fibre for every 100kcal you consume.

✅ **If partially hydrogenated oil,** or trans fats, are listed on the label, step away from the box and protect your health.

✅ **Pick up a jar of dried shiitake mushrooms.** They may look a little strange, but toss them in some hot water for half an hour and you have a meaty, healthy addition to soups, stews and sauces, not to mention a unique filling for tarts and omelettes. Plus, they keep for ages.

▶ **Whenever you find yourself reaching for a packet of minced meat,** go to the poultry section instead and choose minced turkey or chicken, or try Quorn mince. These work just as well as minced beef in, for example, meatballs and chilli. This substitution alone can cut nearly a third of the calories and at least half of the fat and saturated fat in a 85g serving. When it's covered in a zesty tomato sauce or flavoured with seasonings, you won't be able to tell the difference.

✅ **Choose low-fat cheeses.** Instead of high-fat Caerphilly, Cheddar, Double Gloucester or Parmesan, choose ricotta, low-fat cottage cheese or quark. You can also enjoy medium-fat cheeses such as Brie, Edam, Camembert, Danish blue and feta in moderation.

✅ **Buy rapeseed oil instead of vegetable oil.** It's rich in healthy monounsaturated fatty acids and contains the essential fatty acids (EFAs) alpha-linolenic acid (ALNA) and linoleic acid (LA). It also costs less than olive oil.

▶ **Choose wholemeal bread** (sometimes labelled as whole wheat). Studies show that people who eat three or more servings of whole grains a day are less likely to suffer from diabetes. If your family will eat only white bread, choose a fibre-enriched variety.

✅ **Buy plain yoghurt and flavour it at home.** Pre-flavoured yoghurts contain sugars that destroy any healthy benefits. If you add fruit at home, it will still taste yummy, plus you'll consume far fewer useless calories *and* save money.

☺ **Choose healthy toppings for plain cereals.** These include raisins, fresh berries, dried berries, pumpkin seeds and bananas. Buy unsweetened cereals, then add your favourite flavours. That helps you to bypass all the empty sugary calories – and lets you enjoy the cereal more. For ease, keep a wide-brimmed, well-sealed jar of ingredients on your worktop for quick mixing. Have a scoop and some sealable bags handy, and you've got a handy, nutritious meal or snack to eat at home or when you're on the go.

✅ **Read juice labels carefully.** Orange juice, though healthy, often has 20g of sugar in the average 250ml glass. Instead, try guava juice. It has three times more vitamin C and is full of potassium (a great blood pressure regulator) and beta carotene. NB If you have kidney disease or are on a blood pressure-lowering medication, avoid potassium-rich foods as extra potassium may be harmful.

Shiitake mushrooms are a versatile addition to any food cupboard.

Sneaking in
VEGETABLES

The average Brit is lucky to get one serving of vegetables a day, whereas nutrition experts would advise us to eat at least two to three helpings. This is pretty much our health problems in a nutshell. If we ate more vegetables and fewer processed foods, we'd lose weight, clean out our arteries, balance our blood sugar and shut down a large number of hospitals. But getting from one serving a day to three doesn't come without planning or effort. Here's the health-boosting and *painless* way to sneak more veggies into your daily diet.

23 WAYS TO GET YOUR FILL

Fresh or powdered garlic?
ANSWER: **FRESH.**

Technically, the jury is still out. A large American study on fresh garlic by Christopher Gardner, PhD, of Stanford University Medical Center, found that fresh garlic failed to reduce cholesterol levels, although further research is needed on its other possible medicinal benefits. But, Gardner notes, the active ingredient in garlic is allicin, which can easily be destroyed if you mess with it too much, which suggests that fresh is best. Other tests indicate that you'd usually need more powdered garlic than fresh to get the same benefits.

● **Add chopped kale or other hearty greens** to your next soup or stew. Just a couple of minutes is all that's needed to steam the greens down to tenderness and add quantities of potassium, fibre and calcium to your soup.

● **Use low-sodium vegetable juice** as the base for soups instead of chicken or beef broth.

● **Incorporate grated carrots and shredded cabbage in your soups,** salads or casseroles. These coleslaw ingredients add flavour, colour and lots of vitamins and minerals.

☆**Go vegetarian one day a week.** You can do this by merely replacing the meat serving with a vegetable serving (a suggestion: make it a crunchy, strong-flavoured vegetable such as broccoli). Or you can dabble in the world of vegetarian cooking, in which recipes are developed specifically to make a filling, robust meal out of vegetables and whole grains. For those times, you should get yourself a good vegetarian cookbook. Try the *Reader's Digest Vegetarian Cookbook* or *Good Food Magazine's 101 Veggie Dishes*, from BBC Books, for starters.

☺**Use salsa liberally.** First, make sure you have a large batch of tomato salsa filled with vegetables. One good approach: add chopped yellow peppers and courgettes to shop-bought salsa. Then put salsa on everything: baked potatoes, rice, chicken breasts, sandwiches, eggs, steak, even bread. Don't save it just for tortilla chips. It's too tasty and healthy not to be used all the time.

● **Roast your vegetables.** Here's a great side dish that's easy to make, delicious to eat and amazingly healthy. Plus, it tastes surprisingly sweet, and lasts well as a leftover, meaning you can make large batches to serve throughout the week. Cut hearty root vegetables such as parsnips, turnips, carrots and onions into 3cm chunks and arrange in a single layer on a baking sheet. Drizzle with olive oil and sprinkle with sea salt, freshly ground pepper and fresh or dried herbs. Roast in the oven at 230°C/gas mark 8 until soft, for about 45 minutes, turning once.

● **Use vegetables as sauces.** How about puréed roasted red peppers seasoned with herbs and a bit of lemon juice, then drizzled over fish? Why not purée butternut squash with carrots, grated ginger and bit of brown sugar for a yummy topping for chicken or turkey? Cooked vegetables are easily converted into sauces. It just takes a little ingenuity and a blender.

● **Lose the bitterness of healthy veggies with a sprinkle of salt.** There's more about how to reduce the salt in your diet later, but the chemical reality is that salt helps to neutralise bitterness. For an added kick, try capers, olives or mashed anchovies instead of salt.

☺ **Grill your vegetables.** If you use your grill only for meats, you're missing out! Peppers, courgettes, asparagus, onions, aubergine, tomatoes – they all taste great when grilled. Generally, all you need to do is coat them with olive oil and throw them on. Turn every few minutes and remove when they start to soften. Or put chunks on a skewer and turn frequently.

● **Go exotic.** Every week, try to buy a slightly exotic vegetable, perhaps something that you've never eaten before. Here are some ideas, and some preparation and cooking suggestions:

● **Chicory.** This type of lettuce has a mild, slightly bitter flavour, and is packed with fibre, iron and potassium. Use it in salads and with vegetable dips.

● **Bok choy.** An Oriental cabbage, bok choy is excellent chopped and stir-fried in a bit of peanut oil and soya sauce. Or add it to the soup just before serving.

● **Kohlrabi.** A member of the turnip family, this is also called a cabbage turnip. It's sweeter, juicier, crisper and more delicate in flavour than a turnip, and the cooked leaves have a kale/collard flavour. Trim and pare the bulb to remove all traces of the fibrous underlayer just

beneath the skin, then eat the vegetable raw, boiled, steamed, microwaved or sautéed, or add to potato casseroles.

● **Fennel.** Also known as sweet anise, fennel has a mild liquorice flavour. The feathery fronds can be used to flavour soups and stews, while the broad, bulbous base can be eaten raw, or sliced/diced for adding to stews, soups and stuffing.

Counting **TO FIVE**

Learning that you need to get five or more servings of fruit and vegetables a day can be daunting. But consider the definition of a serving below (from the NHS website, www.5aday.nhs.uk), and you'll see that it's perfectly do-able:

● One medium-sized fruit (such as an apple, orange, banana or pear), half a grapefruit, 1 large slice of pineapple, 1 slice of melon or 2 slices of mango.

● 1 tablespoon of dried fruit, such as raisins, currants, sultanas or mixed fruit; 2 figs or 3 prunes.

● 2 broccoli spears, 8 cauliflower florets, 4 heaped tablespoons of kale, spring greens or green beans.

● 3 heaped tablespoons of baked, haricot, kidney, cannellini or butter-beans or chickpeas. (Beans and pulses count as only 1 portion, no matter how many you eat.)

● 3 heaped tablespoons of cooked vegetables such as carrots, peas or sweetcorn (but not potatoes, which don't count at all).

● Salad vegetables such as 3 sticks of celery, 1 medium tomato, 7 cherry tomatoes or a 5cm piece of cucumber.

● One 150ml glass of 100 per cent pure fruit or vegetable juice or smoothie (note that you can count juice as only 1 portion, no matter how much you drink).

Reminder

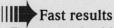 **Fast results**
These are tips that deliver benefits particularly quickly – in some cases, immediately.

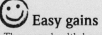 **Easy gains**
These are health boosters that offer the best value for the least amount of effort.

☆ **Super-effective**
This is advice that scientific research or widespread usage by experts has shown to be especially effective.

Sneaking in FRUIT

You've no doubt heard talk of the global economy. Well, you need look no further than your local supermarket to see it in action. There, grapes from South America meet kiwis from New Zealand and pineapples from Hawaii – in February. But because of concerns about the carbon footprint of these items, we are being urged increasingly to buy locally sourced fresh food, which makes sense for good health and for the environment.

You know the drill by now – for optimal health you should be aiming for at least two or three servings of fruit a day. It's not difficult, especially with these clever tips.

21 WAYS TO GET ALL YOU NEED

⭐ **Make it a rule: every breakfast includes a piece of fruit.** It's the ideal morning food, filled with natural, complex sugars for slow-release energy, fibre and nutrients galore. Cantaloupe melon, an orange, berries – all are perfect with wholemeal toast, cereal or an egg.

☺ **Make another rule: eat fruit for dessert at least three nights a week.** A slice of watermelon, a peach, a bowl of blueberries – they're a delicious ending to a meal, and are so much healthier than biscuits or cake. Like more sophisticated desserts? How does chocolate-covered strawberries, poached pears in red wine or frozen fresh raspberry yoghurt sound? They count too.

🍈 **Every Monday, start your week with a fruit 'slushie'.** Add 160g of fresh fruit, 125ml of fruit juice and a handful of ice cubes to a blender and liquidise. That gives you two servings of fruit before 8am. If you'd prefer a creamier smoothie, add 125ml of plain fat-free yoghurt.

🍈 **Substitute fruit sorbet for ice cream.** One scoop contains up to one serving of fruit.

🍈 **Keep a fruit bowl filled wherever you spend the most time.** This could be at work, near your home computer or even in the television room. And keep five to eight pieces of fresh fruit in it at all times, such as bananas, oranges, apples, grapes or plums. Most fruit is fine left at room temperature for three or four days. But if it's out and staring at you, it's not likely to last that long.

🍈 **Carry dried fruits with you.** Dried fruits are very portable and have a long shelf life. Take them to work, on shopping trips or even on holiday. Raisins and

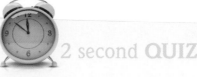
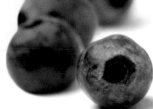

prunes are classic choices. Also try dried cranberries and blueberries, which are extremely high in phytonutrients, or dried apricots, which are chock-full of beta carotene. Other options include dates and dried figs, peaches, pears and bananas.

☺ **Take fruit with you whenever you are driving for more than an hour.** Once you're on the motorway and cruising along, an apple or a nectarine tastes great and helps to break the tedium.

🍈 **Keep an apple in your pocket** whenever you go for long walks. It will be your reward for getting to the midpoint of your chosen route.

🍈 **Make Monday red day.** And eat only red fruits. Tuesday could be orange day and so on. Here's how your weekdays might work to give you maximum fruit variety (you could make weekends a fruit free-for-all):
Monday. Red: apples, cherries, cranberries, red grapes, plums, strawberries.
Tuesday. Orange: apricots, cantaloupe melon, kumquats, nectarines, oranges, papaya, peaches.

Fresh fruit or dried?
ANSWER: **FRESH.**

The higher water content (most fresh fruits are more than 80 per cent water) means a larger volume, making the fruit more filling and satisfying with fewer calories. But for convenience and shelf life, use dried fruit as your back-up plan.

Wednesday. Yellow or white: bananas, yellow apples, grapefruit, mango, pineapple.
Thursday. Blue or violet: blackberries, blueberries, grapes, plums, figs.
Friday. Green: limes, pears, green apples, kiwi fruits.

Mix fruits in with your salad. A sprinkling of raisins, some chopped strawberries, a diced apple, some fresh or dried mango or some sliced kiwi all make tasty additions to the typical tossed salad.

Purée fresh or canned fruits (peaches, pear, mangoes, apricots, etc.) and use as a delicious and healthy ice cream or pancake topping.

Add frozen berries to cereal, salads or ice cream. They also work well stirred into yoghurt or muffin mix.

Freeze banana slices or grapes for a refreshing summer snack. Simply pop the banana slices and/or grapes into a sealable bag, freeze, then eat as desired.

Every time you want a chocolate bar, eat a small box of raisins instead. Raisins are sweet and healthy, and small boxes contain just the right amount to fulfil the need for a sweet treat.

Get your fruit from bread and cake once a week. How about apple cake, banana bread, strawberry, apple or blueberry tart? Pineapple upside-down cake, anyone?

Spice up shop-bought salsas with fruit. Or make your own fruit-based salsas with pineapple, mango or papaya. Mix with onions, ginger, a bit of garlic, some mint and/or coriander, sprinkle on a few hot pepper flakes for a bit of a kick, and enjoy.

Add diced kiwi, sliced grapes or chopped apple to chicken, tuna and turkey salads.

Keep cubed or sliced melon in a container in the fridge. Use as a first course before dinner; wrap with prosciutto for a starter; mix with cottage cheese for breakfast; have a small bowl for a snack; even consider puréeing it for a quick sauce over fish.

Grate fruit over plain yoghurt. Use the larger holes of a box-type grater for a quick and tasty topping.

Mash bananas and spread them on toast and bagels for a treat that brings back childhood. Or freeze whole bananas for a delicious, healthy summer snack.

Every week, buy one exotic fruit you've never tried. It could be something as relatively common as a mango, or as unusual as a cherimoya. Here are some tips on some exotic fruits and how to enjoy them:
● **Asian pear.** Also called an Oriental, Chinese, salad or apple pear, this firm pear is meant to be eaten immediately when it's hard. It's sweet, crunchy and amazingly juicy.

- **Cherimoya.** Also called a custard apple, this large tropical fruit tastes like a combination of pineapple, papaya and banana. Purchase fruit that's firm, heavy for its size and without skin blemishes or brown splodges. Let it soften at room temperature, then refrigerate it, wrapped, for up to four days. To serve, cut it in half, remove the seeds and spoon the fruit from the shell.
- **Guava.** Sweet and fragrant with bright pink, white, yellow or red flesh. Buy when it is just soft enough to press, and refrigerate it for up to a week in a plastic or paper bag. To use, cut in half and scoop out the flesh for salads, or peel and slice. Try cooking and puréeing slightly underripe guava as a sauce for meat or fish.
- **Kiwi fruit.** This fruit didn't take off until its name was changed from Chinese gooseberry to kiwi fruit. Now it's one of the most popular of the exotic fruits. With a flavour that's a cross between strawberries and melon, kiwis are ready to eat when they're slightly soft to the touch. Peel and chop, or cut in half and scoop out the flesh with a grapefruit spoon.
- **Lychee.** Once, lychee trees were found only in southern China, but the popularity of this tropical fruit has caused its spread. The lychee fruit is about 4cm in size, oval, with a bumpy red skin. Peel off the inedible skin and you get a white, translucent flesh similar to a grape, but sweeter, surrounding a cherry-like stone. Eat them like large grapes, one after another. They're available for only a few months of the year, but buy a bag in spring and you'll discover why Asian people call lychees the king of fruits.
- **Mango.** Until relatively recently, mangoes were not widely available in UK supermarkets. But in the wider world, they're one of the most commonly eaten

In PERSPECTIVE

Deconstructing antioxidants

The reason that fruits (and vegetables) are so important to your overall health is that they are major purveyors of antioxidants. Antioxidant molecules are like the missile-defence system of your body, preventing damage from molecular bombs called free radicals. It works like this: in order to breathe, move or eat, your body's cells convert food and oxygen into energy. This chemical reaction releases harmful by-products, the free radicals. Basically, they are highly reactive forms of oxygen that are missing an electron. Desperate for that missing electron, they steal them from normal cells, damaging the healthy cell and its DNA in the process. This damage eventually contributes to any number of major health problems, including heart disease, memory loss and cancer.

Antioxidants, however, interfere with this process by giving free radicals one of their own electrons to stabilise them. Or they combine with free radicals to form different, more stable compounds. There are also antioxidant enzymes that help free radicals to react with other chemicals to produce safe, instead of toxic, substances. Antioxidants, for instance, help to prevent 'bad' LDL cholesterol from becoming stickier and forming artery-clogging plaque.

This is why the health establishment is so insistent on people eating more fresh produce: it provides round-the-clock defences against free-radical damage to your arteries.

Guava makes a great sauce for meat or fish.

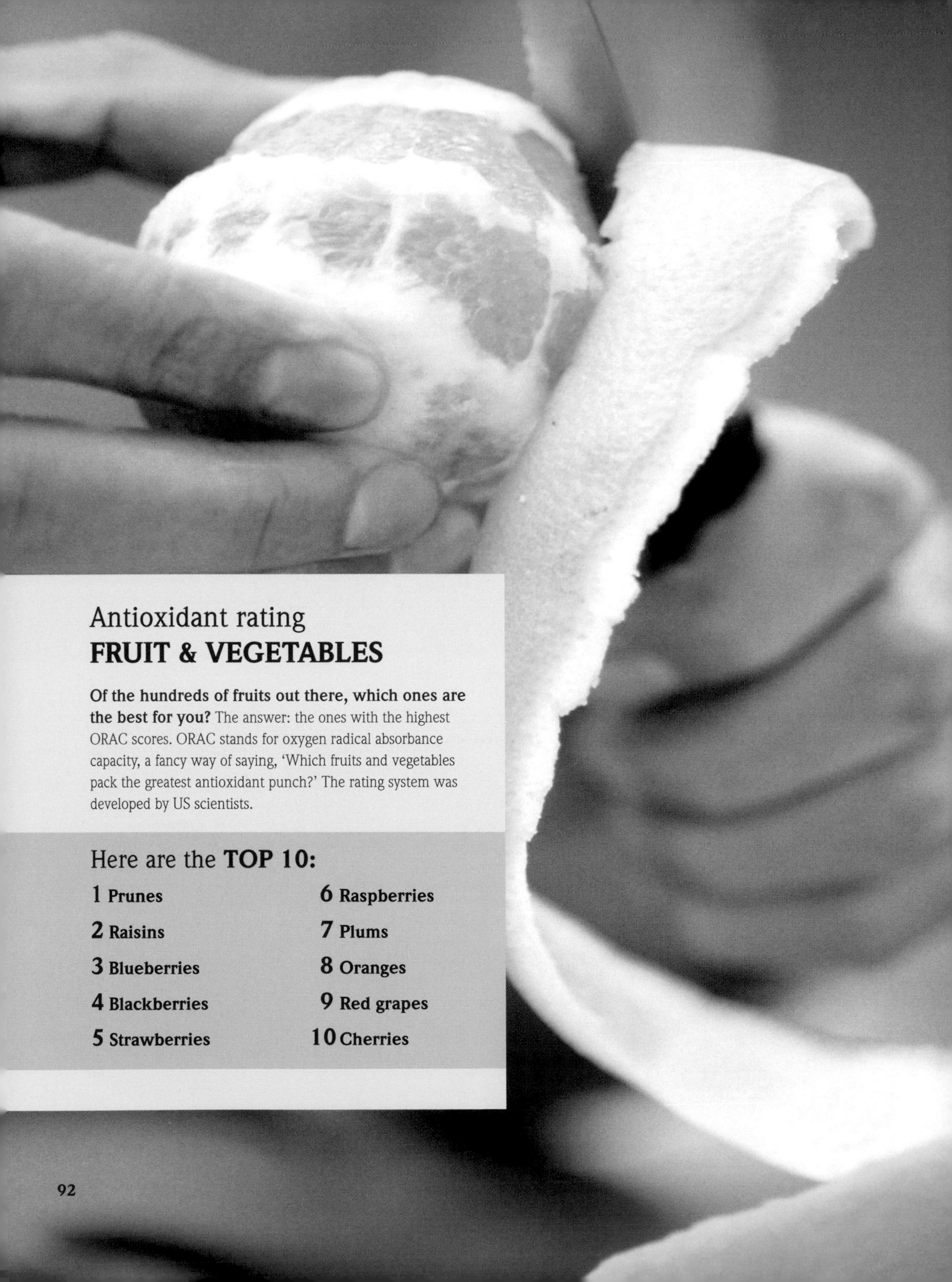

Antioxidant rating
FRUIT & VEGETABLES

Of the hundreds of fruits out there, which ones are the best for you? The answer: the ones with the highest ORAC scores. ORAC stands for oxygen radical absorbance capacity, a fancy way of saying, 'Which fruits and vegetables pack the greatest antioxidant punch?' The rating system was developed by US scientists.

Here are the TOP 10:

1 Prunes

2 Raisins

3 Blueberries

4 Blackberries

5 Strawberries

6 Raspberries

7 Plums

8 Oranges

9 Red grapes

10 Cherries

fruits, along with bananas. The flavour is a combination of peach and pineapple, but spicier and more fragrant (it is sometimes called the tropical peach).

● **Papaya.** Soft, juicy and silky-smooth flesh with a delicate, sweet flavour. The centre of the papaya is filled with small, round, black, pepper-tasting seeds, which can be eaten but aren't usually. Peel, then slice into wedges or cut into chunks, or slice in half, remove seeds and scoop out the flesh with a spoon. Unripe papayas can be peeled, seeded and cooked as a vegetable, and you can grind the seeds like pepper for adding to sauces or salads.

● **Passion fruit.** Passion fruit has golden flesh with tiny, edible black seeds and a sweet-tart taste. When ripe, it has wrinkled, dimpled, deep purple skin. To serve, cut in half and scoop out the pulp with a spoon.

● **Persimmon.** Delicate in flavour and firm in texture, the persimmon, sometimes called the Sharon fruit, can be eaten like an apple, sliced and peeled, and is great in salads.

● **Pomegranate.** Available in the autumn, it's the seeds of this crimson fruit that you eat. Each tiny, edible seed is surrounded by translucent, brilliant-red pulp that has a sparkling sweet-tart flavour. Choose fruit that feels heavy for its size with a bright colour and blemish-free skin. Pomegranates can be refrigerated for up to a month, while the seeds can be frozen for three months. To serve, cut the fruit in half and prise out the seeds. Use them to top ice cream, sprinkle into salads or eat simply as a snack.

● **Quince.** Tastes like a cross between an apple and a pear, with a dry, hard, yellowish-white flesh that has a tart

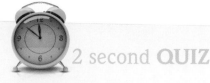
flavour. Better cooked than raw. Quinces keep for up to two months wrapped and refrigerated, and are primarily used for jams, jellies and preserves.

● **Star fruit.** Slice crossways for perfect five-pointed star-shaped sections as a garnish or as an ingredient in fruit salads. The star fruit's flavour combines the best of plums, pineapples and lemons.

● **Tamarillo.** This subtropical fruit is sometimes called a tree tomato, but the comparison ends there. Native to South America, this egg-shaped fruit has a glossy outer skin that hides crimson fruit which turns golden when cooked or heated. The orange-yellow flesh, studded with a swirl of edible dark-red seeds, has the texture of a plum and is slightly tart. To peel tamarillos, plunge into boiling water for about 30 seconds, then slip off the skins. Cut crossways into slices.

Pomegranates are packed with jewel-like seeds bursting with flavour.

Sneaking in **FIBRE**

The term 'good' carbs refers to complex carbohydrates. These are foods, such as whole grains and beans, which are composed largely of complex sugar molecules that require lots of time and energy to digest them into the simple sugars your body needs for fuel. One of the biggest benefits of these foods is that they also contain large amounts of fibre – the indigestible parts of plant foods. Fibre protects you from heart disease, cancer and digestive problems. Depending on the type of fibre, it also lowers cholesterol, helps with weight control and regulates blood sugar. This is one nutrient you don't want to miss. Yet the average person in the UK gets just 12g to 15g of fibre a day – far below the recommended 24g. In the next two chapters, we'll talk about how to remove 'bad' carbs from your diet and up your 'good' carbs – two of the best things you can do for your health.

25 WAYS TO GET MORE 'GOOD' CARBS INTO YOUR DIET'

● **Enjoy cereal every day for breakfast.** Ideally, aim for a whole-grain, unsweetened cereal with at least 3g of fibre a serving. Just eating any cereal might be enough, though. A University of California study found that cereal eaters tend to eat more fibre and less fat than non-cereal eaters.

● **Eat two apples every day.** Not just to keep the doctor away, but because apples are a good source of pectin, a soluble fibre that contributes to a feeling of fullness and which is also digested slowly. A 1997 study published in the *Journal of the American College of Nutrition* found that 5g of pectin was enough to leave people feeling satisfied for up to 4 hours.

▐▐▐➡ **Designate one day a week to have a yoghurt mix for breakfast.** Take one pot of yoghurt and mix in 30g of All-Bran cereal, 1 tablespoon of ground linseeds and 5 large, diced strawberries for a whopping 12.2g of fibre – half your daily needs.

☺ **Mix your usual cereal with the high-fibre stuff.** You might not want to face an entire bowl of All-Bran in the morning. But a 30g serving contains a massive 8g of fibre. Mix it with an equal amount of your usual cereal and you'll barely know it's there (but you will be a third of the way to your daily fibre intake).

● **Dip baby carrots and broccoli florets into low-fat yoghurt dip or salsa** for your afternoon snack three days a week. You'll fill up the empty afternoon space in your stomach while getting about 5g of fibre from each 150g of veggies.

● **Make sure that the first ingredient in whole-grain products has the word 'whole' in it,** as in 'wholemeal' or 'whole grain'. If it says multigrain, seven-grain,

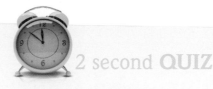

2 second QUIZ

Broccoli or cauliflower?
ANSWER: **BROCCOLI.**

At 2.6g of fibre per 100g, broccoli has twice the fibre oomph of cauliflower.

nutragrain, cracked wheat, stone-ground wheat, unbromated wheat or enriched wheat, it's not wholemeal, and is thus lacking some of the vitamins and minerals, not to mention fibre, of whole grains.

● **Keep a snack container in your car and office for the munchies.** Mix together peanuts, a high-fibre cereal such as All-Bran and some chocolate-covered raisins. Allow yourself one handful for a sweet, yet high-fibre, snack.

● **Switch to rye crackers.** You'd never think a tiny cracker could make a difference, but two standard cream crackers contain 0.4g of fibre, while two rye crackers have 2.3g of fibre.

● **Add kidney beans or chickpeas to your next salad.** A 100g serving of kidney beans, for example, contains 8g of fibre.

▐▐▐➡ **Every week, try one 'exotic' grain.** How about amaranth, bulghur or wheatberries? Most are as simple to prepare as rice, yet are packed with fibre and flavour. Mix in some steamed carrots and broccoli, toss with olive oil and a bit of Parmesan or feta cheese, maybe throw in a can of tuna or 50g or so of sliced chicken, and you've got dinner.

Eat two apples a day. And not just to keep the doctor away.

In PERSPECTIVE

The weight-loss wars

For a while now, there has been a war among both consumers and doctors regarding the best approach to weight loss: a low-carbohydrate diet or a low-fat diet. In terms of popularity, the winner is clear: low-carb diets such as Atkins have won the hearts of many weight-conscious people. But the medical establishment remains vehement about the low-fat message. So why can't they all just agree?

As is often the case, research has caught up with all the claims, and proved that there are strengths and weaknesses in both approaches. The message is that excess animal fat in your diet is indeed bad for your health and your weight. But certain fats, particularly plant-based fats such as olive oil, are necessary for good health and nutrition. Likewise, excessive amounts of simple carbohydrates are bad for your health too. They are converted too easily into blood sugar, and cause all types of metabolic havoc when you eat them regularly. Much better are unrefined, whole-grain foods that take longer to digest and contain more nutrients and fibre.

Put it all together and you get a sensible diet rich in complex carbohydrates and lean, healthy meats and seafood. Plus loads and loads of vegetables.

At the end of the day, weight loss is about eating moderate amounts of healthy foods. What had been confirmed most recently is that simple carbs are more unhealthy than was once thought. Respond sensibly to that finding, and you are on your way to a lifetime of healthier eating.

Or serve as a side dish to chicken or fish. Make sure all the grains you try are whole grains.

● **Once a week, make pearl barley** (which doesn't require any soaking before cooking) as a side dish. A 100g serving of cooked pearl barley contains 3.8g of fibre.

☺ **Sneak in oatmeal.** Use basic oatmeal in place of breadcrumbs for meatballs, sprinkle it on top of casseroles and ice cream, bake it into biscuits and muffins, and add it to homemade bread and cakes.

☺ **Use wholemeal bread to make your lunchtime sandwich every day.** Even sandwich shop chains offer wholemeal options for lunchtime munching. If you want to break into the wholemeal club gradually, use wholemeal bread as the bottom slice of your sandwich and white bread as the top layer. Eventually, make the move to all wholemeal.

● **Every week, switch from a white food to a brown food.** So instead of instant white rice, you switch to instant brown rice. Instead of your usual pasta, choose wholemeal pasta. Similarly, go for wholemeal pittas and wholemeal couscous. Within two months, you should be eating only whole grains, and you should have increased your daily fibre intake by an easy 10g without radically changing your diet.

● **Spread your sandwich with hummous.** Add 2 heaped tablespoons of hummous and you've got 2g of tasty fibre. Add some spinach leaves and a tomato slice for another couple of grams.

● **Make beans a part of at least one meal a day.** They're packed with fibre (9g per 100g) and, since they come canned, they're user-friendly. Just rinse first to remove excess salt. Here are some health-boosting tips for getting your beans:
● Purée a can of cannellini beans for a tasty dip. Add 2 cloves of garlic and a tablespoon each of lemon juice and olive oil to the blender. Use as a dip for veggies and whole-grain crackers.
● Fry a couple of tablespoons of mixed beans with some onion and chicken in a little oil and use to fill a soft flour tortilla.
● Mix black-eyed beans with finely chopped onion, chilli, garlic and tomatoes to make a salsa.
● Make a bean salad with canned black-eyed beans, fresh or frozen sweetcorn,

chopped coriander, chopped onion and chopped tomato. Drizzle with olive oil and a dash of vinegar, salt and pepper.

● Make your own special chilli pizza. Top a prepared (wholemeal) pizza base with some kidney beans, grated cheese and minced turkey cooked with chilli.

● Start serving edamame (soya beans) as a side dish. You'll get 5g of fibre from 100g of edamame, not to mention the cancer-fighting phytonutrients that soya contains.

● **Add puréed cauliflower to mashed potatoes.** You won't taste much of a difference, but you'll get some extra fibre.

● **Have a beetroot salad for dinner.** These bright red veggies have virtually no fat, no cholesterol, no sodium, quite a bit of potassium and 2g of fibre. Try roasting whole, peeled beetroots for 45 minutes, chilling, then dicing into a summer salad.

● **Make rice pudding for dessert tonight.** Only, instead of white rice, use brown to kick it up a notch.

● **Switch to wholemeal flour when baking.** You can start by going half and half, eventually using only wholemeal for all your cooking needs. Adding a little baking powder helps to lighten foods made from wholemeal flour (note that you may have to add a little more liquid if using wholemeal flour).

▐▐▌➤ **Add some linseeds, wheatgerm** or other high-fibre ingredients to batter. They add crunch to your biscuits, muffins and breads – and loads of fibre.

● **Eat the skin of your baked and sweet potatoes.** Eating baked potatoes with the skin on ups the fibre by at least 3g (depending on the size of the potato).

Do **THREE** things...

The three best ways to get more fibre into your diet:

1 Eat more fruit and vegetables. They're the healthiest fibre sources around.

2 Start each day with a bowl of whole-grain cereal.

3 Switch to a whole-grain bread.

● **Start every dinner with a mixed green salad.** Not only will it add fibre, but, with a low-calorie dressing, it will partially fill you up with very few calories, and thus offers great weight-loss benefits.

● **Use beans or lentils as the main protein source** for dinner once or twice a week. A classic dish such as pasta e fagioli (pasta with beans) works well.

● **Drink your fibre.** Make your own smoothies by blending whole fruits (take out the large pips or seeds). If all the fruit goes into your glass, you'll get all the fibre – often missing from fruit juice.

DON'T FORGET to ...

Drink plenty of water. You need water to help the fibre pass through your digestive system without getting stuck. So as you're increasing the fibre in your diet, also increase your intake of water or other unsweetened drinks. And don't up your fibre intake all at once. That's just going to overwhelm your system, leading to gas, bloating and constipation. Instead, start slowly. Try one tip a week for the first couple of weeks, then two, then three. By week four or five, you should be up to the full 24g – or more.

Cutting back on
'BAD' CARBS

Thanks to the popularity of low-carb diets, many of us are now watching the amount of carbohydrates we eat. The last chapter detailed the benefits of 'good' carbs. Now it's time to explain what a 'bad' carb is. Put simply, it's white flour, refined sugar and white rice. More broadly, it's any carb that has been processed to strip out ingredients which hinder quick and easy cooking. Why are refined carbs a problem? Easy: they are digested so quickly that they cause blood sugar surges, leading to weight gain and other health troubles. The next chapter shows you ways to reduce the amount of sugar you eat. For now, read on for other ways to avoid troublesome carbs while still getting enough fuel for good health.

10 WAYS TO AVOID THE WORST CULPRITS

● **Say no to the bread basket.** At almost every restaurant, the first thing a waiter brings is a basket of rolls and bread made from white flour. If it's not put on the table, you won't eat any. Or, if you really need something to nibble on, ask if they have wholemeal varieties.

● **Choose brown rice, not white,** and limit how much you eat to 180g. Brown rice hasn't been processed and it still has its high-fibre nutrients.

☺ **Wrap your food in lettuce leaves.** Yes, skip the rolls, tortillas and bread slices and instead make a sandwich inside lettuce leaves. Go Mexican with a sprinkle of Cheddar cheese, salsa and chicken; or Chinese with sesame seeds, peanuts, bean sprouts, sliced green beans and prawns with a touch of soy sauce; or deli style with turkey, cheese and mustard.

● **Buy your snacks in child-sized bags.** The truth is, crisps, tortilla chips and biscuits are mostly bad carbs, made primarily from refined flour, sugar, salt and/or oil. You want to remove as many of these foods from your daily eating as you can. But if you can't live without them, buy them in small bags – 30g is a typical 'lunch box' size – and limit yourself to one bag a day.

▰▰▶ **Cure yourself of your old spaghetti habits.** Almost everyone loves a big bowl of pasta, topped with a rich tomato sauce. The tomato sauce couldn't be better for you; the spaghetti, however, is pure carbohydrate. While spaghetti is fine to eat every now and then, for those sensitive to carbs or wishing to cut back on their pasta intake, here are some alternatives to the usual spaghetti dinner:
● Here's the easiest choice: switch to wholemeal pasta. It's denser than

traditional pasta, with a firm, al dente texture similar to what you'd get in Italy.
● Grill vegetables such as aubergines, courgettes, peppers and onions and slice into long, thin pieces. Mix up and pour your spaghetti sauce over the vegetables for a tasty and immensely healthy meal.
● Try healthy whole grains as a replacement for pasta. Spaghetti sauce goes better than you'd expect on brown rice, barley, chickpeas and so on.

Cutting the carbs without HITTING YOUR WALLET

Specialist low-carb diets can be expensive. For easy ways to stay low-carb without breaking the bank, follow these recommendations:
● Replace salmon and other more expensive fish with chicken breast or tofu.
● Always buy frozen fish rather than fresh (much fresh fish has been previously frozen anyway). There is little nutritional or taste difference, but you will see savings in price.
● Buy frozen berries, including blueberries, strawberries and raspberries. They're almost always less expensive than fresh (except maybe during peak growing season for your area).
● Replace mixed green salads with any dark leafy green (mustard, kale, spinach). Buy whole heads of greens rather than bagged and washed greens, which could cost up to 20 per cent more.
● Replace extra virgin olive oil on salads and in recipes with lower grade olive oil or rapeseed oil.

In PERSPECTive

Glycaemic index vs. glycaemic load

The glycaemic index (GI) is a measure of how much, and how fast, the sugar in a food raises the level of sugar in your blood. A high or fast rise in blood sugar leads to high blood insulin levels, contributing to weight-control problems and possibly even increasing your risk of diabetes over time. So, in theory, a high glycaemic index is a bad thing.

But the measure has important limitations. For one thing, it compares foods directly to one another to determine which raises blood sugar more. These comparisons are based on an equivalent 'dose' of sugar in each food in an effort to be fair. To make the dose of sugar in carrots equivalent to the dose of sugar in ice cream, however, calls for the comparison of a tiny dish of ice cream to a bushel of carrots. Of course, the carrots will have the higher glycaemic index. It's also based on the effects of just one food, eaten alone. In real life, the foods we eat interact with each other to determine blood sugar levels. High-fibre cereal at breakfast, say, will blunt the rise in blood sugar from eating high GI foods at lunch.

A newer measure, the glycaemic load, accounts for both how fast the sugar in a food is converted to blood sugar and the dose of sugar in the food. Whereas the glycaemic index of a fizzy drink is similar to that of carrots, the glycaemic load of the fizzy drink is ten times higher than that of carrots.

Should you worry about the glycaemic index or load of the foods you eat? That's one for your doctor to answer. If you have diabetes or are prone to blood sugar swings and weight gain, being aware of the impact of food on your blood sugar is important. But for most of us, a healthy diet probably precludes the need to track these measurements.

● **Cut up 30g portions of cheese** and measure out 30g portions of nuts, then put one of each into snack bags. Now you have a handy snack at the ready.

● **Eat potatoes boiled with the skin still on.** The effect of potatoes on blood sugar depends on how the potatoes are prepared. There's no need to avoid them completely, but keep your portion size modest. Also, new potatoes tend to have fewer simple carbs than other types of potatoes.

▌▌▌➤ **Never let yourself get too hungry.** Eat every 3 to 5 waking hours, and only until you're satisfied but not stuffed. You should never reach the point where you feel ravenous. Not only is that a recipe for overeating, but your body will want sugary, quick-to-digest 'bad' carbs to satiate your need for fuel quickly.

● **Instead of eggs and bacon, try a bowl of porridge.** Sweeten it with sugar-free sweetener or sugar-free muesli.

● **At the cinema, skip the popcorn.** Popcorn isn't a bad food – it contains useful fibre, for example. But it does happen to be a simple carb with little other nutritional value and, when bought at the cinema, it's often drowning in salt and fat. Better snacks are small bags of nuts or seeds and fresh or dried fruit. Just take them into the cinema with you.

Porridge is a tasty high-fibre way to start the day.

Cutting down on SUGAR

Britain is drowning in sugar. In fact, in the past two decades, British sugar consumption has increased by 31 per cent, to more than half a kilo per person per week. Although fewer of us take sugar in our tea, and we sprinkle less on our cereals and puddings, we are actually consuming more, hidden away in processed foods, leading to weight problems and obesity. Even worse, as sugary foods often replace more healthy foods, nutrition experts say the influx of sweets indirectly contributes to diseases such as osteoporosis, heart disease and cancer – all of which are directly affected by what we eat. In this third chapter on carbohydrates, there's advice on getting your sugar consumption down to healthy levels.

20 WAYS TO GET RID OF THE SWEET STUFF

Don't have ice cream tempting you in the freezer. If you want some of this sweet treat, go out and buy it.

● **Cut down slowly.** Forget going cold turkey. Therein lies failure. Instead, if you normally have two chocolate bars a day, cut down to one. Then, next week, have one every other day. The following week, have one every three days, until you're down to just one a week. If you normally take 2 teaspoons of sugar in your coffee, use the same routine, cutting down gradually to ½ teaspoon. Eventually, get to the point where you're using artificial sweetener if you still need the sweet taste. The more sugar you eat, the more you'll crave. So cutting down slowly is the best way to tame a sweet tooth gone wild.

● **Choose sugar-free and reduced-sugar alternatives** to foods such as baked beans, ketchup and cereals, when available.

● **Go half and half.** Mix half standard fizzy drink with half diet version; half a pot of sweetened yoghurt with half a pot of plain yoghurt; half a glass of juice with half a glass of fizzy water. Do this for two weeks, then cut back to a quarter sweetened to three-quarters unsweetened. Continue until you're taking only the unsweetened version.

● **Grant yourself a daily sugar 'quota',** and use it on the foods where it matters most. For the majority of us, that means desserts. Don't waste it on dressings, spreads, breakfast cereals and fizzy drinks. Not only will this reduce your sugar intake in a day, but it will help you to lose your sweet tooth. The more sugar you eat, the less sensitive your taste buds seem to become, so you want more. Train your taste buds to become accustomed to less and you'll be satisfied with less.

▐▐▐► **Establish rules about dessert.** For instance, have dessert only after dinner, never after lunch. Or eat dessert only on odd days of the month, or just at weekends or in restaurants. If you have a long tradition of daily desserts, then make it your rule to have raw fruit at least half of the time.

● **Similarly, establish rules about ice cream.** A tub of ice cream in the freezer is temptation defined. A recommended rule: no ice cream kept at home. Ice cream should always be a treat worth travelling for.

▐▐▐► **Remember these code words found on ingredient lists.** The only way to know if the processed food you're buying contains sugar is to know its many aliases or other forms. Here are the common ones: brown sugar, corn syrup, dextrin,

2 second QUIZ

An apple or sugar-free apple sauce?
ANSWER: **AN APPLE.**

You'll get all the nutrients of the apple sauce, but you'll also get the added fibre kick from the skin of the apple, which is removed before the apple sauce is made.

dextrose, fructose, fruit juice concentrate, high-fructose corn syrup, galactose, glucose, honey, hydrogenated starch, invert sugar, maltose, lactose, mannitol, maple syrup, molasses, polyols, raw sugar, sorghum, sucrose, turbinado sugar.

● **Try xylitol.** Xylitol is a natural sweetener as well as a sugar substitute, which is found in fruits such as strawberries, pears and plums. It is very like sugar in appearance, so is often added by manufacturers to sweets and chewing gums, as well as to medicated syrups and some mouthwashes and toothpastes. It's safe for those with diabetes and it actually improves the quality of your teeth, as well as having fibre-like health benefits. Beware, though: eating large quantities of xylitol may have a laxative effect.

● **Look for hidden sources of sugar.** Cough syrups, chewing gum, mints, tomato sauce, baked beans and cold meats often contain sugar. Even some prescription medicines contain sugar. For a week, be particularly vigilant and scan every possible food label. Make a mental note of what you discover.

● **If you must eat sweets, eat them with meals.** The other foods will help to increase salivary flow, thus clearing the sugary foods from your mouth faster and helping prevent cavities. Of course, this does nothing for the calories you're imbibing and won't affect your weight, but at least you'll have a healthier mouth.

● **Seek out substitutes.** With saccharin, aspartame, accsulfame potassium and sucralose all commercially available, you can still get the sweetness of sugar without the calories. These sweeteners can be particularly useful as part of a diabetic diet.

In PERSPECTIVE

Corn syrup

Ask people what they think of when they hear the word 'sweet', and chances are they'll reply 'sugar'. But since its arrival in the marketplace in 1966, the real story in the sweetness world has been corn syrup, to the point that some newspapers and magazines are now declaring this alternative sweetener to be the number one evil in our diets. High-fructose corn syrup is generally cheaper and easier to refine than granulated sugar. So, increasingly, processed-food companies have been switching to corn syrup to add sweetness to their products, especially in soft drinks and juices. That would have been the end of the story, except for recent research results which suggest that the human body processes corn syrup differently from sugar.

According to the studies, when the body processes sugar, it triggers the production of a chemical that signals fullness to your brain, and also prevents the release of a chemical that indicates hunger. But when scientists monitored how the body processes corn syrup, the worst-case scenario seemed to have occurred: the hunger chemical wasn't affected, and the fullness chemical was suppressed. In short, corn syrup, in theory, makes you hungrier.

Is this true? Doctors are debating the point. Many believe that the issue is merely that calories consumed as liquid are less filling than calories from solid food, independent of the form of the calories.

Whatever the case, corn syrup is a big issue for anyone trying to eat healthily. It is a huge source of empty calories that mess with your body's chemistry. So fight back, starting with any drinks that you buy. If corn syrup is one of the main ingredients in a drink, put it back.

● **Substitute apple sauce or puréed prunes for half the sugar in recipes.** You can also use them in place of the fat in the recipe.

☺**Choose the right breakfast cereal.** Many are full of sugar. You want one with less than 8g of sugar per serving or, preferably, one that is unsweetened altogether. Use diced fruit instead to sweeten your cereal.

Dip fresh strawberries in a low-fat chocolate sauce for a decadent treat.

● **Don't skip meals.** Are you too busy to eat? When you go without breakfast, lunch or dinner, your blood sugar levels drop, and that propels you towards high-sugar (often convenience) foods to quell your cravings.

● **Don't add sugar to foods.** Many everyday recipes – including some for vegetables, soups, casseroles and sauces – call for sugar to add sweetness. In most cases, it's just not needed. Try the recipe without the sugar first. If you think it needs sugar after tasting, you can always add it, but don't do it automatically.

● **Get your chocolate in small doses.** Dip fresh strawberries into low-fat chocolate sauce, scatter chocolate sprinkles over your plain yoghurt or eat a mini-piece of dark chocolate – freeze it so that it lasts longer in your mouth. Think rich and decadent but in tiny portions.

● **Watch out for mixed alcoholic drinks.** Have you ever stopped to think about the sugar quotient of a cosmopolitan? How about a margarita or mai tai? Drink mixers and many alcoholic beverages are absolutely thick with sugar. Stick with beer, wine or, if you prefer spirits, mix them only with unsweetened fizzy water or drink them straight. Of course, a glass of fizzy water with lime will also do just fine.

☆ **Go for a walk when you crave sweetness.** Studies find that athletes' preference for sweetened foods declines after exercise. Instead, they then prefer salty foods.

● **Choose fat-free if you must have sweets.** Studies find that many sweet foods, such as doughnuts, muffins, ice cream and so on, are also high in fat, more than doubling the calorie load. When you do indulge in sweet foods, choose fat-free options, so you get the full flavour of a favourite food with none of the calories from the added fat.

● **If you're having a hard time cutting back on fizzy drinks or juices,** try having a glass of iced water or fizzy water every other time you reach for a drink.

2 second QUIZ

Brown sugar or white sugar?
ANSWER: **NEITHER.**

They're both sugar. Neither has any nutritional benefit or is any better than the other. Here's a case where the brown colour does not imply a healthier version.

Cutting back on
'BAD' FATS

We've come a long way from the days when all fat was bad. Today, researchers have identified 'good' fats (monounsaturated and polyunsaturated) and 'bad' fats (saturated and trans fats). So we can now eat certain fats and still be perfectly healthy. The down side? You have to be conscious of four types of fats. But there's an easy way to work it out: basically, if a fat is solid at room temperature – animal fats, butter, lard, some nut oils – chances are it's a bad fat. The good fats are usually found in fish and plant oils, but even they have their limits. All fats provide your body with 9kcal per gram, more than twice as much as proteins or carbohydrates. For good health, keep your total fat intake to 30 per cent of calories or less and your saturated fats to less than 10 per cent. Trans fats? Keep them to zero.

27 WAYS TO GET LEAN THE RIGHT WAY

Cutting back on **SALT**

Ask anyone about salt and they'll tell you it's bad for you. They're wrong. Salt is not bad for you. Salt (sodium chloride) is essential to your well-being and you need about 1.4g a day to keep your body ticking over. What's bad is excessive salt or, actually, the sodium part of salt. The average salt consumption in the UK is about 9g a day, most of it from processed foods. Experts, who recommend an intake of no more than 6g a day, have calculated that if we reduce our salt intake by around 2.5g a day, it would reduce the risk of having a stroke or heart attack by a quarter. Not only that, a high-salt diet can have other adverse effects such as osteoporosis, stomach cancer and obesity, as well as exacerbating asthma symptoms. So try these tips to make food taste great without all that shaking going on.

17 WAYS TO EAT WELL WITHOUT IT

● **Invest in a pepper mill.** Use freshly ground black pepper instead of salt, or look out for lemon pepper, a seasoning that adds wonderful flavour, not salt, to foods.

● **Mix low-salt foods with standard foods** to start you on the path to reducing your salt intake. For instance, mix unsalted peanuts with salted. Slowly increase the amount of the salt-free product as you decrease the amount of the salted until you're eating only the salt-free version.

● **Say no to sports drinks.** Research does indicate that endurance athletes need higher levels of salt and far more to drink than everyday folk. Sports drinks deliver both – they are rich in salt, which not only provides the necessary sodium but also stokes continued thirst. For the rest of us, the extra salt provides no benefit at all. Even if you exercise regularly, unless you are testing your body's physical limits for extended periods, water should be fine to quench your thirst.

● **Keep your table salt in a small bowl,** and use a tiny spoon or a pinch of your fingers to season your food. You'll find that you use far less of it. Cover it with a snug lid or some clingfilm to keep it dry (and make it less accessible).

● **Put a big X on your calendar for six weeks from today.** Unlike our preference for sugar, which we're born with, salt is an acquired taste, learned from habit. So it takes time to 'unlearn' your preference – about six weeks, to be exact. Slowly reduce your intake of salt between now and then, focusing on food categories where the salt will be missed the least, such as cereals, breads and dessert items. As long as you know you aren't going to stop wanting salty food overnight, you won't get discouraged.

SODIUM and SALT

Salt is also called sodium chloride. It's the sodium in salt that can be bad for your health. Sodium is usually listed in the nutritional information on food labels. Salt is also listed on some foods, but not all.

Salt = sodium x 2.5. If you know how much sodium is in a food, you can work out roughly the amount of salt it contains by multiplying the sodium by 2.5. So if a portion of food contains 1.2g of sodium, it contains about 3g of salt.

How can I tell if a food is high in salt?

Here's a quick way to tell if a food has a high salt content by checking the nutritional information on the label. Look at the figure for salt per 100g.
● **High is** more than 1.5g of salt per 100g (or 0.6g of sodium).
● **Low is** 0.3g of salt or less per 100g (or 0.1g of sodium).
● If the amount of salt per 100g lies somewhere between these figures, it contains a medium level of salt.

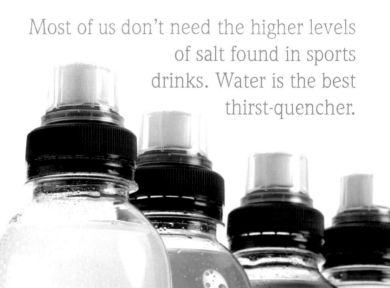

Most of us don't need the higher levels of salt found in sports drinks. Water is the best thirst-quencher.

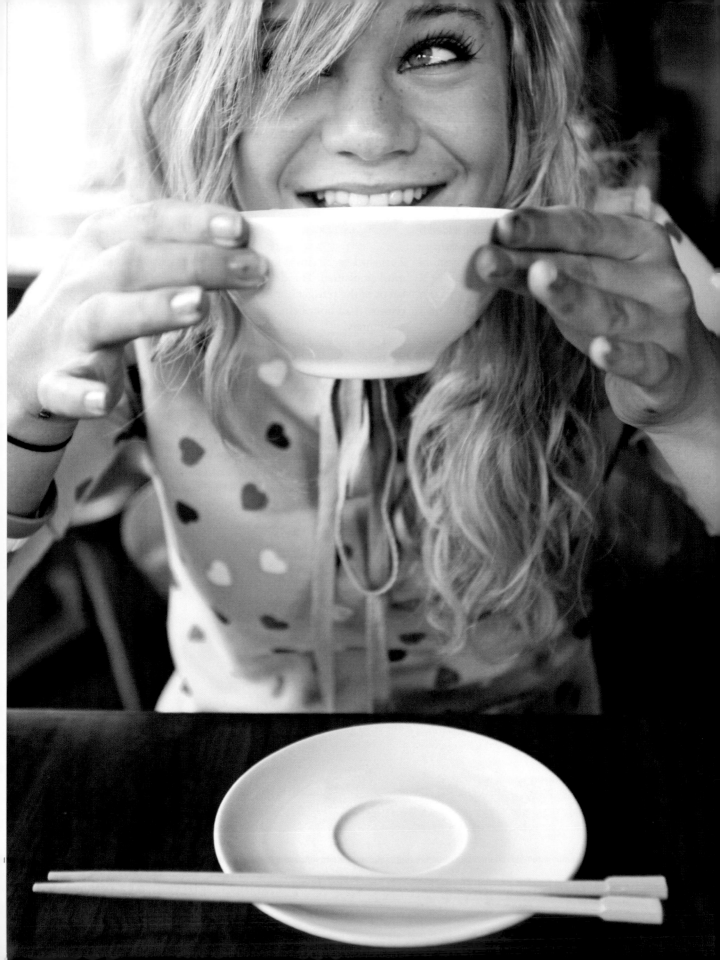

part 3

DINING OUT

Eating healthily at home is an excellent first step. But for all-round healthy eating, you need to control what you eat when you're not at home. Here's the best advice.

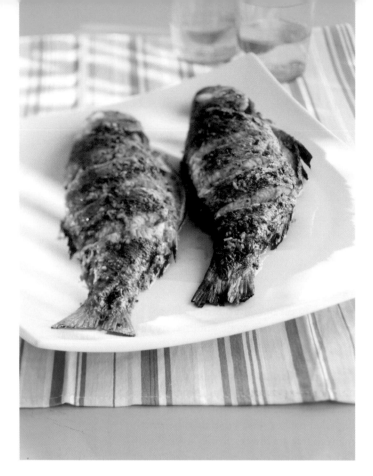

Have your fish any way but fried.

whopping 560kcal, with 36g of fat, 6 of them saturated. Italian antipasto salads are also a health challenge, with all their salami, spicy ham and cheese. Get the salad, but ask for vegetables only.

Do the fork dip. The best way to combine salad dressing with salad? Get your dressing on the side, in a small bowl. Dip your empty fork into the dressing, then skewer a forkful of salad. You'll be surprised at how this tastes just right, and how little dressing you'll use.

Top a baked potato with veggies from the salad bar. Or ask if you can have salsa – the ultimate potato topper, both in terms of flavour and health. Just avoid the butter and soured cream.

Check out the menu before you leave home. Most chain restaurants post their menus on their websites. You can decide before you even open the door what you're going to order. Conversely, if you don't see anything that's healthy, pick another restaurant.

Read between the lines. Any menu description that uses the words creamy, breaded, crisp, sauced or stuffed is likely to be full of hidden fats – much of it comprising saturated or even trans fats. Other words to beware of include: buttery, sautéed, pan-fried, au gratin, thermidor, Parmesan, cheese sauce, scalloped, as well as au lait and au fromage (with milk and with cheese).

Don't assume that ordering vegetarian will be the lower-calorie choice. It isn't always the case – avoid dishes containing lots of nuts and cheese, for example.

Ask the waiter to skip the bread basket. If you must have something to munch on while you wait for your meal, ask for a plate of raw vegetables or some breadsticks.

Avoid the fancy drinks. If you insist on ordering an alcoholic drink, forget the margaritas, piña coladas and other exotic mixed drinks. They include sugary additions that pile on the calories. Opt instead for a glass of wine, a light beer, a vodka and tonic or a simple martini.

Order fish. But make sure it's not fried. Fish is a good low-fat, low-salt option. Plus, you can order seafood cooked so many different ways – steamed, baked, barbecued, sautéed, blackened or grilled. Avoid any sauce, or ask for it on the side.

Drink water throughout the meal. It slows you down, helps you to enjoy the food more, and gets the message to your brain that you're full – before your plate is empty. If it doesn't come automatically, ask for a jug of water as you sit down.

Keep an eye on your wine glass refills. If you're drinking wine, don't allow the waiter to fill up your wine glass before it's empty. If your glass is constantly being topped up, it's impossible to keep track of how much you've had to drink.

Always dress up to go out, even if it's to an ordinary family restaurant. If you view eating out as an event or a treat, rather than as a way to get an everyday dinner, you won't eat out as often. And that's good from both a health and a cost point of view.

Skip the dessert. You can always have some sorbet or even a small piece of chocolate at home. That is much more healthy than a rich chocolate Black Forest gateau or a mountain of ice cream topped by a second mountain of whipped cream. Plus, it will save you money.

Cuisine-specific advice

A perk of modern living is having so many restaurants to choose from. But with choice comes confusion. To help, here are tips for sensible eating at some of the most popular restaurant types.

Health-boosting British dining means you:
● Leave the batter. Fish and chips are not a great choice, but if you really can't resist, leave the batter and eat the fish inside. Also limit yourself to ten chips. Fish cakes are a better choice, but avoid any creamy hollandaise sauce.

DEADLY SECRETS
of the restaurant trade

How do restaurants make their food taste so good? Here is the unhealthy truth:

● **BUTTER** In the soup. In the sauce. On the meat. On the vegetables. Butter is the easiest, quickest way to make dishes taste rich and wonderful.

● **OIL AND FAT** Another way to make foods taste richer is to use lots of oil (remember, oil is a fat). This is why fried foods taste good: they're sponges for the oil in which they're cooked. Then there's animal fat. Want to make anything taste better? Add bacon or other forms of pork fat – to vegetables, soups and mashed potatoes.

● **SALT** When you cook at home, you may shake in a little salt as you go. At a restaurant, it's poured in to give maximum flavour.

● **SWEETENERS** Ever have vegetables that tasted sweeter than a dessert? That's because the cook added lots of sugar.

● Avoid pies or anything with pastry. Shepherd's pie or casseroles are better alternatives.
● Eat a small steak. Steak is a good choice, but go for a small one and ask for it to be served with vegetables, salad or a jacket potato rather than chips.
● Keep an eye on the cooking method. Look out for dishes described on the menu as chargrilled, steamed, poached or grilled, all of which are lower in fat.

Health-boosting Chinese dining means you:
● Order fewer dishes than there are people at the table. Chinese starters are designed for sharing, not for one person.
● Start with soup to fill you up.
● Avoid fried starters. So no spring rolls. And have dumplings steamed, not fried.
● Also opt for steamed rice, not fried. If the restaurant serves brown rice, go for it.

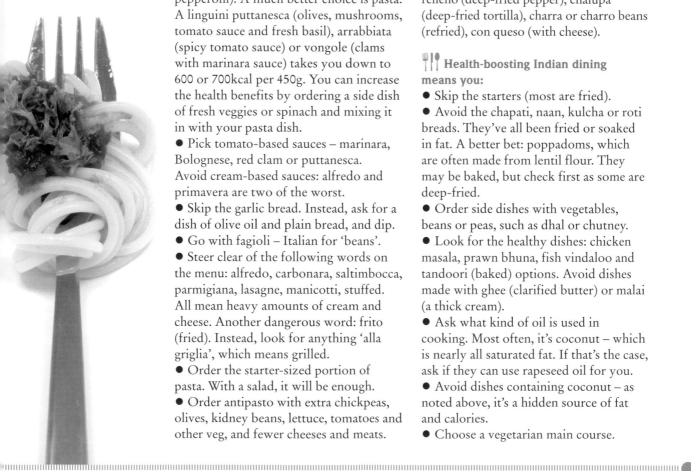

- Use the 2:1 ratio. Eat twice as much rice as main dish.
- Avoid menu items described as crispy, golden-brown or sweet-and-sour. They're all deep-fried.
- Choose dishes rich in vegetables and order at least one vegetarian starter.
- Eat with chopsticks. You'll get less of the high-calorie, high-salt sauce that way.

Health-boosting Italian dining means you:

- Split and share. One order of pasta is usually enough for two people, especially if you also have a salad.
- Dine on pasta rather than pizza. Pizza dough is calorie-dense – about 275kcal per 100g (without the cheese, sausage and pepperoni). A much better choice is pasta. A linguini puttanesca (olives, mushrooms, tomato sauce and fresh basil), arrabbiata (spicy tomato sauce) or vongole (clams with marinara sauce) takes you down to 600 or 700kcal per 450g. You can increase the health benefits by ordering a side dish of fresh veggies or spinach and mixing it in with your pasta dish.
- Pick tomato-based sauces – marinara, Bolognese, red clam or puttanesca. Avoid cream-based sauces: alfredo and primavera are two of the worst.
- Skip the garlic bread. Instead, ask for a dish of olive oil and plain bread, and dip.
- Go with fagioli – Italian for 'beans'.
- Steer clear of the following words on the menu: alfredo, carbonara, saltimbocca, parmigiana, lasagne, manicotti, stuffed. All mean heavy amounts of cream and cheese. Another dangerous word: frito (fried). Instead, look for anything 'alla griglia', which means grilled.
- Order the starter-sized portion of pasta. With a salad, it will be enough.
- Order antipasto with extra chickpeas, olives, kidney beans, lettuce, tomatoes and other veg, and fewer cheeses and meats.

Health-boosting Mexican dining means you:

- Keep away from the fried tortilla chips. Instead, ask for a few soft tortillas to scoop up the healthy salsa and help you to get a couple of vegetable servings under your belt straight away.
- Pick beans to fill your burritos instead of beef or cheese.
- Choose fajitas. Not only can you fill up on the vegetables, but you can pick and choose how much cheese to add.
- Ask for black or pinto beans, not refried.
- Avoid the soured cream.
- Go for soft tacos, not hard tacos. Hard taco shells are fried; soft shells are baked.
- Avoid dishes with the following words in their names: chimichanga (fried burrito), relleno (deep-fried pepper), chalupa (deep-fried tortilla), charra or charro beans (refried), con queso (with cheese).

Health-boosting Indian dining means you:

- Skip the starters (most are fried).
- Avoid the chapati, naan, kulcha or roti breads. They've all been fried or soaked in fat. A better bet: poppadoms, which are often made from lentil flour. They may be baked, but check first as some are deep-fried.
- Order side dishes with vegetables, beans or peas, such as dhal or chutney.
- Look for the healthy dishes: chicken masala, prawn bhuna, fish vindaloo and tandoori (baked) options. Avoid dishes made with ghee (clarified butter) or malai (a thick cream).
- Ask what kind of oil is used in cooking. Most often, it's coconut – which is nearly all saturated fat. If that's the case, ask if they can use rapeseed oil for you.
- Avoid dishes containing coconut – as noted above, it's a hidden source of fat and calories.
- Choose a vegetarian main course.

Dine on pasta rather than pizza.

TAKEAWAY food

Here in Britain we eat more fast food and takeaways than any other European country. As a nation, we consume a mighty 2 billion takeaways a year. Some are healthy, others less so; if you stick to double cheeseburgers, large chips and fizzy drinks, you could see your waistline expand rapidly and your cholesterol levels soar. But something has been happening to fast-food restaurants. As we have become more concerned about what we eat, the KFCs, McDonald's, Burger Kings and many others have taken notice. They've added salads that actually fill you up, reduced serving sizes and introduced more healthy dishes. Here's how to take advantage of these changes, and how to choose the best dishes from some of the UK's many takeaway restaurants.

17 WAYS TO MAKE THE RIGHT CHOICE

● **Go for the salad, minus the fried toppings.** Although most fast-food restaurants offer decent-sized salads these days, if you top them with fried chicken, cheese and the entire contents of the dressing packet, you will end up with as much artery-clogging saturated fat and calories as if you'd had the double-cheeseburger and fries (we often say 'calories' but kcal or kilocalorie, which you see on food labels, is the technically correct term). Instead, choose grilled or roasted chicken as your protein source, skip the croutons and ask for the low-fat dressing – then use only half.

● **Skip the cheese.** Craving a burger? That's OK – just get a plain burger without the cheese. For instance, at McDonald's that saves you 50kcal, 40 of them from fat, and 2g of saturated fat.

☺ **Ask for extra onions, lettuce and tomato.** Whatever sandwich you choose, it'll now be healthier, crunchier and more filling. And it ticks off one more serving of vegetables from your day's quota.

● **Order water.** Or if you must have a fizzy drink, choose the diet version. A large coke contains 210kcal. Making this one change might save you the same number of calories as the meal you're about to eat.

A tasty, filling potato, in its jacket, is a great fibre provider.

☆ **Always say no to the 'special' sauce.** Many are just dressed-up mayonnaise, and thus overflowing with fat and calories. The best topping for your chicken, fish or burger? Mustard (few calories, lots of flavour). The second best? Ketchup (no fat, but a fair amount of sweetener). Other good choices: olive oil and vinegar (in moderation), spicy sauces, red pepper sauce.

● **Do not supersize.** Ever. Even McDonald's is now phasing out some of its supersized items.

● **In fact, order a child's meal.** A small burger, a small fries and an orange juice is a surprisingly filling meal for most adults, and has many fewer calories than the adult version. Plus, you get a free toy!

☺ **Give sweet-and-sour dishes a wide berth.** These meals should be a rare treat – one portion may contain as much as 8 teaspoons of sugar. That includes lemon chicken and some spicy beef dishes. Chicken with cashew nuts or peppers, stir-fried noodles and seafood dishes are all healthier, especially if you have boiled rice or noodles rather than egg fried rice.

● **Look for ways to sneak in fibre.** That means a baked potato (with skin on) and chilli (no cheese), bean burritos and tacos instead of meat (a bean burrito has 12g of fibre – roughly half your daily needs met) and baked beans and corn on the cob (without butter) as side (or main) dishes.

● **Stay away from coconut milk.** Some cuisines, such as Thai, use a lot of coconut milk as a base, which is high in saturated fat. You'll leave the takeaway shop healthier if you opt to start with a soup such as tom yam, beef or chicken satay or Thai fish cakes, and follow up with a chicken, pork or fish-based noodle dish. Thai menus often feature lots of delicious vegetarian dishes too, as well as salads.

● **Try a drier style of curry.** Some of the drier Indian dishes, such as Tandoori, tikka and bhuna, are usually the lower-fat options on the menu. Other healthier choices include vegetable and shellfish-based curries and dishes such as sag aloo (spinach and potato) and mutter paneer (peas with cheese) and baltis. It goes without saying, avoid anything deep-fried.

 Go for skinless chicken, particularly when you're eating at KFC. Ditch the skin – and much of the batter – and you'll save 240kcal and 16g of fat.

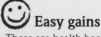 **Choose chicken, not doner.** Research by Dr Tom Sanders, Professor of Nutrition at King's College London, showed that of nine types of takeaway foods tested, a doner kebab was the outright loser. These kebabs were found to contain far more trans fats than any other takeaway meal. If you fancy a kebab, choose a chicken skewer instead, and pile on the salad.

● **Look for the words 'grilled', 'baked' or 'chargrilled'.** If something's cooked that way, it's not fried – and you'll automatically be reaping some savings in terms of fat and calories.

Healthy **INVESTMENT**

A box of cereal bars
Try the crunchy type – more substantial and pleasing to eat – and splash out on a whole box, which could cost the same as a large combo meal at a fast-food restaurant. Keep them in the car as a preventive measure against impulse visits to fast-food places. Next time your stomach growls when you're driving down a takeaway-filled high street, have a cereal bar instead. Then have a healthy meal at home.

● **Have an apple, banana or fat-free yoghurt,** or some other healthy snack an hour before you go for your takeaway. That way you won't arrive starving.

☺ **Make a supermarket your fast-food restaurant.** Run in, grab a piece or two of fruit, a pot of yoghurt, an energy bar, a salad at the salad bar, a turkey sandwich at the deli counter, and you'll be out via the express check-out with breakfast, lunch and snacks in 10 minutes.

● **Avoid processed or cured meats.** That includes hot dogs, salami and ham. These heavily processed meats are often full of fat, salt, chemical additives and, in some cases, sugar. At a deli or a sandwich shop, go for turkey breast, chicken breast or roast beef instead.

Reminder

▶Fast results
These are tips that deliver benefits particularly quickly – in some cases, immediately.

☺**Easy gains**
These are health boosters that offer the best value for the least amount of effort.

✩**Super-effective**
This is advice that scientific research or widespread usage by experts has shown to be especially effective.

READY meals

These days, many of us stop at the supermarket on our way home, not for raw ingredients for supper but for ready-prepared, 'home-cooked' meals that just need to be slipped into the microwave for a few minutes. They're called 'ready meals', and more and more supermarkets are turning over large sections of floor space to them, as well as to frozen foods. If you're willing to spend the money, you may never need to cook or eat at home again (in fact, it's estimated that the average British man now gets a quarter of his food energy intake from food eaten outside the home, while women get 21 per cent). As with everything in life, though, what you choose helps to determine your health. Here are a few basic guidelines for shopping wisely for food, wherever you are.

12 WAYS TO MAKE THEM AS HEALTHY AS HOME COOKING

● **If you buy pre-prepared food to save time,** buy only those things you don't have time to make. The less you buy pre-made, the more control you have over what you're eating. So choose a rotisserie chicken, by all means, but also go to the fresh food department for a potato to microwave instead of buying fried or roast potatoes, and add some broccoli that you can quickly steam or some colourful fresh salad ingredients.

☺ **Always think vegetables.** How are you going to get vegetables into your meal? If you don't want to cook, fill a salad bar container with raw veg, but stay away from too many marinated veggies. And, of course, those pre-washed mixed greens make salad preparation about as complicated as finding a bowl. But remember that it's always better and tastier to prepare your own from fresh.

☺ **Get two meals at a time.** Again, you're trying to save time. So that whole roasted chicken you got for tonight can double as a chicken Caesar salad tomorrow night. If you're making a bowl of couscous to go with your takeaway dinner tonight, double the amount and pick up some extra vegetables and feta cheese at the salad bar for a Mediterranean salad the following night. Or perhaps for lunch tomorrow.

● **Go for sushi.** Low in fat, sushi is one of your best bets when running into your supermarket for dinner, and many shops now stock a good selection. Can't stand the thought of raw fish? Lots of shops offer cooked-fish sushi or even veggie-only sushi.

● **Grab a can of beans before you pay for your food.** Then add the beans to the salad bar selection you've just bought.

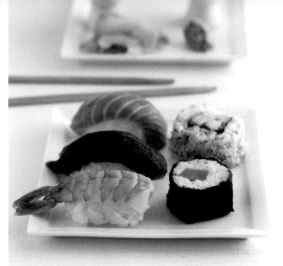

Be good to yourself: choose fresh sushi from your supermarket.

You'll save money (because beans are so filling) while still adding valuable fibre and other nutrients to the salad.

▶ **Have an indoor picnic for dinner.** For a fresh take on healthy eating, buy a loaf of whole-grain bread, a punnet of strawberries, a favourite low-fat cheese, some thinly sliced roast beef or turkey, a small tub of olives, pre-cooked prawns,

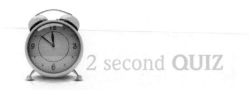

2 second **QUIZ**

Soup or salad?
ANSWER: **SALAD.**

Of course, some soups are far healthier than some salads. But, in general, you're better off with a salad of mixed greens and raw vegetables, coupled with a light, healthy dressing. You'll get more fibre and thus more filling for your calories, not to mention the healthy dose of disease-fighting antioxidants found in raw vegetables. Many soups are very healthy, but the cooking process can diminish some of the ingredients' nutritional value.

Health-boosting **PIZZA**

In the UK we spend £748 million each year on takeaway and home-delivery pizzas; the chain Domino's alone sold us almost 37 million pizzas in 2008. Although it's not the healthiest food you could choose, there's no reason to cut pizza out of your life – it offers a quick, easy, tasty way to get loads of vegetables, fruit, fibre and even fish. But pizza, like any other takeaway/ sit-in food, has its own pitfalls. When American scientists evaluated pizza slices from the top chains, it discovered fat levels approaching – and sometimes surpassing – a fast-food cheeseburger. The main culprit: far too much cheese. Add to that fatty meat such as sausage and pepperoni, and you are in the unhealthiest reaches of the food world. Here's how to make pizza a healthy delight:

- Order half-fat cheese or no cheese.
- Ask for extra veggies.
- Steer clear of stuffed-crust pizzas. You don't need the extra cheese.
- Avoid anything called Meat Lover's, All the Meat or Super Supreme. In fact, order your toppings individually.
- The best toppings: after veggies and fruit (ever tried pineapple-topped pizza?) come chicken, ham, prawns and anchovies. These offer the greatest nutritional punch with the lowest saturated fat.

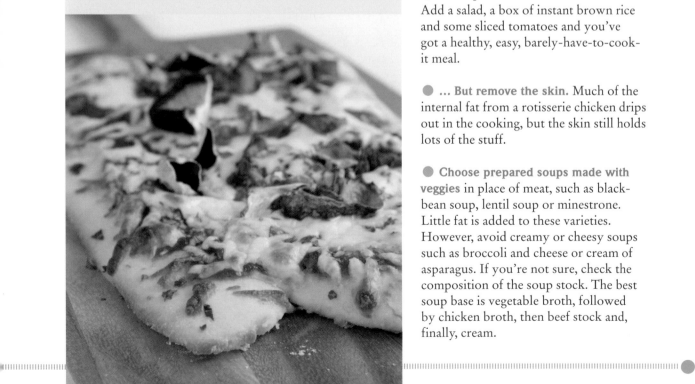

cherry tomatoes, pre-sliced green or red peppers and bite-size carrots. When you get home, throw it all on the table and – after properly cleaning any fruit or veg – declare that dinner is served. This type of 'grazing' dinner is fun, easy and a pleasant change. Make it a twice-monthly ritual.

● **Order sandwiches or rolls with turkey or chicken,** lots of vegetable fillings such as tomato, lettuce, peppers and cucumber and just a little spread. Ask for whole-grain bread.

● **Order twice as much** of the prepared vegetables as you do of the main course.

● **If you can see that there's mayonnaise** pooling around the chicken, tuna, seafood or pasta salads, skip them. Mayonnaise is a combination of eggs and oil – primarily fat.

● **Pick up a rotisserie chicken …** Add a salad, a box of instant brown rice and some sliced tomatoes and you've got a healthy, easy, barely-have-to-cook-it meal.

● **… But remove the skin.** Much of the internal fat from a rotisserie chicken drips out in the cooking, but the skin still holds lots of the stuff.

● **Choose prepared soups made with veggies** in place of meat, such as black-bean soup, lentil soup or minestrone. Little fat is added to these varieties. However, avoid creamy or cheesy soups such as broccoli and cheese or cream of asparagus. If you're not sure, check the composition of the soup stock. The best soup base is vegetable broth, followed by chicken broth, then beef stock and, finally, cream.

PICNICS

Eating outside in the sun, with the crash of waves on the beach or the wind through the trees as your musical accompaniment, makes any meal taste better. That's why picnics should feature in your healthy-eating master plan. If the word 'picnic' is synonymous in your mind with overstuffed sandwiches, potato salad and crisps, this is for you. Here are 13 health-boosting ways to ensure that dining al fresco doesn't translate as dining al fatso!

13 WAYS TO GO BEYOND SANDWICHES AND POTATO SALAD

COFFEE shops

What would the world be like without Starbucks and other coffee shops? Somewhat thinner, perhaps. These havens for coffee lovers, specialising in sweet drinks to wash down irresistible pastries and cakes, have become a staple in the UK and elsewhere – there are 15,000 Starbucks around the world. That's not counting all the smaller chains and local coffee shops. What's worrying is that they're a major, often hidden, source of fat and calories. Did you know that a Starbucks Java Chip Frappucino made with whole milk and whipped cream has more calories and saturated fat than a McDonald's Quarter Pounder with cheese? Read on to find out how to make coffee shop visits healthier.

9 WAYS TO GET OUT HEALTHY

☕ **Classify pastries as treats, not breakfast.** A pastry as an occasional treat is fine, but as a breakfast it's disastrous. Not only will the simple carbohydrates and high sugar leave you drooping and hungry an hour later, but you get little to no nutritional benefit from the fat and calories. If you must eat on the run at your coffee shop, order a wholemeal bagel.

☺ **Classify speciality coffee drinks as dessert, not coffee.** Fancy-flavoured, whipped-cream, hard-to-pronounce coffee drinks can be worse for you than a big slice of cake. For example, a medium Java Chip Frappuccino with whipped cream at Starbucks has 510kcal, 22g of fat and 59g of sugar. Of the various cakes, muffins and pastries Starbucks lists on its website, most have fewer calories per serving than the drink. If you must have a fancy coffee drink, treat it like a banana split or a cake – a rare indulgence, to be had by itself and not as a mere beverage.

☕ **Choose biscotti.** These twice-baked Italian delicacies are perfect for dunking; at Starbucks they carry just 110kcal and 5g of fat.

☺ **Order plain coffee and add the extras yourself.** Not only are many of the speciality coffee drinks at coffee shops loaded with fat and calories, but some items are made from mixes, some of which may contain large amounts of trans fats. The solution: get a black coffee and add in healthy amounts of skimmed milk, sugar or sugar substitute and, if you wish, top with separate flavourings such as ground chocolate or cinnamon.

☕ **If you must order speciality beverages,** order those made with milk, such as cappuccino or latte. And ask that they be made with skimmed milk. You'll

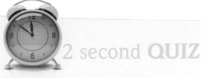

2 second QUIZ

Starbucks café au lait or caffe latte
ANSWER: **CAFÉ AU LAIT.**

Café au lait comprises equal parts brewed coffee and steamed milk. A caffe latte is one or two shots of espresso with steamed milk and foam filling the rest of the cup. For a tall drink made with semi-skimmed milk, the au lait has just 91kcal and 3.4g of fat, while the tall semi-skimmed latte, because it uses so much more milk, has 148kcal and 5.6g of fat. You may find that the au lait has a bolder, more coffee-rich flavour, so you win on all counts.

get a good amount of calcium along with the warmth and caffeine but without the saturated fat.

☕ **Forget the whipped cream topping.** You'll instantly save 100kcal and 10g of fat.

☕ **Share a muffin with a friend.** As with a pastry, think 'treat' rather than breakfast when you order a muffin at a coffee shop. Muffins – even bran muffins – tend to be more about good-to-taste than good nutrition.

☺ **Go for a flavoured bagel.** If you're ordering blueberry, cinnamon and raisin or some other tasty flavour, you won't need the extra cream cheese, butter or other spreads. Better still, go for wholemeal, multigrain or oat-bran varieties – you can eat your bagel and have some good nutrition too.

☕ **Pick the low-fat option.** Many coffee shops and bakeries do offer low-fat versions of their tasty treats. This is still a long way from health food, but it's a health-boosting step closer.

Fruit bagels are tasty without the spreads.

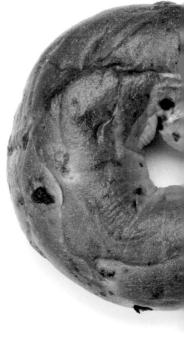

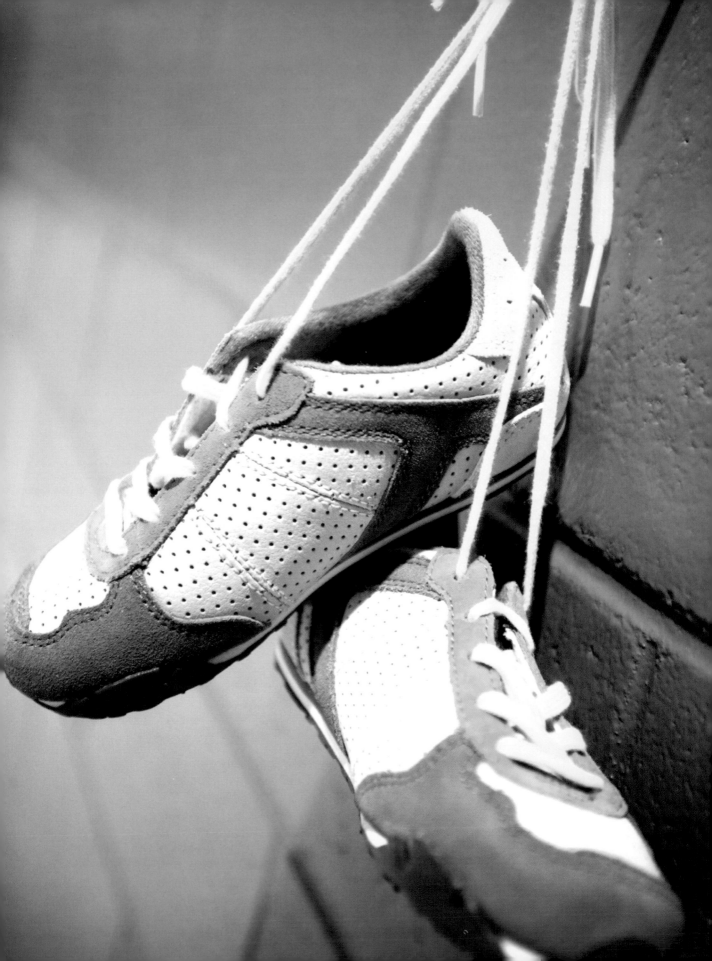

part 4

HEALTH BOOSTING EXERCISE

After tackling food, there's no better way to improve your health than by getting up and moving. Here's how to work extra movement into your days without hassle or sweat.

STRETCHING

The human body was engineered for standing and moving. Sitting all day long – as so many office workers and TV viewers do – is unnatural, and takes its toll on our well-being. To survive the daily office-job marathon without eventually suffering some form of chronic pain or injury, it's important to stretch regularly. Of course, stretching is good for more than just that. One of the most common complaints about ageing, for example, is stiffness and joint pain. Stretching regularly helps to keep you lithe, active and injury-resistant. And a regular stretching routine may even improve your sleep. The following 14 tips will show you how to sneak some stretches into your day.

14 WAYS TO SNEAK IN SOME LIMBERING UP

EARLY MORNING routine

● **Every morning, roll out of bed and do these stretches.**
Can you get away with just three stretches for your entire body? 'Yes, if your main goal is overall body health,' says Claire Small, specialist musculoskeletal physiotherapist and co-founder/director of London-based Pure Sports Medicine, a sports, medicine and high-performance centre. Small suggests the following gentle mini-routine first thing in the morning just after getting out of bed. It's safe to perform even with cold muscles.

1 TRUNK EXTENSOR STRETCH Prepare your back for the challenge of sitting at a desk all day long with this stretch, above. Repeat it periodically during the day to release tension in your lower back. Sit on the floor with your knees bent and feet flat on the floor. Lift your toes until only your heels touch the floor. Sit tall with your back straight and spine long and extended. Place your hands on your shins. Tuck your chin into your chest, bend forward from the hips, and pull your torso as far down as you can. Hold for 2 seconds, release, then repeat ten times.

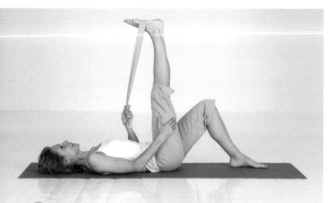

2 HAMSTRING STRETCH This will help to lengthen your hamstrings first thing in the morning.

Lie on your back with your knees bent and your feet on the floor. Lift your right knee in towards your chest and thread a rope (or a tie or towel) round the arch of your right foot. Hold the ends of the rope with your left hand. Extend your leg towards the ceiling. Place your right palm against your right thigh and press into it as you use the rope to increase the stretch. Hold for 30 seconds, release and repeat three times. Switch legs and repeat.

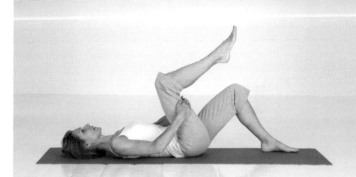

3 PELVIC TILT Doing this stretch helps to increase blood flow to your midsection, relaxes your back muscles and helps to realign your sacrum, one of the large, flat bones that form your pelvis.

Lie on your back with your knees bent and feet on the floor. Lift your right thigh towards your chest, grasping the back of your thigh with both hands. Bring your knee as close to your chest as you can. Hold for 2 seconds, release, then repeat ten times. Switch legs and repeat.

● **Stretch during your shower.** The perfect time of day to squeeze in a little stretching is right after – or during – a warm shower in the morning. 'Your muscles are warm and it's a great way to energise your day,' says David Smith, Strength Conditioner for Worcester Rugby Club. He suggests trying the following routine:

● While in the shower, raise your arms above your head, clasp your hands and reach upwards to stretch your shoulders and back.

● With the water spray hitting the back of your neck, slowly turn your head to the right until your chin is over your shoulder. Pause, then slowly turn your head all the way to the left. Repeat five times in each direction.

● Dry off with one foot on the edge of the bath or shower tray, lean forward and stretch your hamstring.

● While drying your hair, hold a calf stretch by extending one leg 0.5 to 1m behind the other.

● **And get in some stretching with each bite of breakfast.** Do this sitting down. As you eat, roll your ankles in clockwise and anticlockwise circles. Then draw large, imaginary letters with your big toes, spelling your first, middle and last name with each foot.

||||▶ **Better still, do a more thorough 3 minute stretching routine every morning.** This routine works for two reasons: first, it comprises very simple, natural moves; second, it is particularly good for anyone with stiff joints or mild arthritis. It gently warms your muscles and moves your shoulders, knees, elbows, wrists and neck through a full range of motion, stimulating the release of synovial fluid, a thick secretion that lubricates and cushions your joints. Complete the following stretches from a standing position, starting with whatever range of motion you feel comfortable with and gradually increasing it as your joints warm up. Complete 10 to 12 slow repetitions of each stretch, moving clockwise and anticlockwise, pausing for a moment at the full extension on each stretch.

Neck roll. Bring your chin to your chest, then move your chin in a half-circle, bringing your left ear over your left shoulder, then your right ear over your right shoulder.

Shoulder shrug. Lift your shoulders to your ears, then slowly drop them.

Shoulder circle. Slowly roll your shoulders in circles.

Arm circle. Extend your arms straight out to your sides, so they are parallel to the ground. Slowly whirl them in circles as if they were propellers on an aeroplane.

Hip circle. With your knees slightly bent and your feet placed slightly wider than your hips, circle your hips in one direction and then the other, as if you were balancing a hula hoop.

● **Do finger stretches regularly to keep your hands nimble and strong.** Do one hand at a time for best effect.

Finger stretch. Place a hand on a tabletop or thigh, with your palm facing down. Spread your fingers as far as you can and hold for 20 to 30 seconds.

Thumb touch. Place your hand, palm up, on a table with your fingers open and relaxed. In a smooth movement, touch the tips of your thumb and index finger together. Hold this for a second, then return to the starting position. Then touch the tip of your thumb to all of your other fingertips.

Spider walk. Place your hand palm-down on a tabletop. Use your fingers to pull your palm across the table as far as you can reach.

Good stretching TECHNIQUE

Follow these tips to increase the effectiveness of your stretching routine:

● **Feel the muscle you are targeting.** As you slowly proceed through the movement, you should feel a stretching sensation in your muscle as it lengthens and relaxes. If you feel a sharp pain in a joint, such as your knee, you have either gone too far or your technique is at fault. If you feel nothing at all, you have either not gone far enough or, again, are using the wrong technique.

● **Relax.** Many people tense up as they stretch, for example, hunching their shoulders towards their ears. Don't. Notice whether you are clenching any other muscles and gently allow them to release as you exhale.

● **Breathe into it.** If you breathe slowly and deeply as you stretch, you'll increase blood flow and make your stretching more effective. Always exhale as you move into the stretch. As you hold, inhale by expanding the abdomen, ribcage and chest, then exhale as you visualise your breath flowing through the tension you feel in your muscle.

● **Stretch each and every day.** When it comes to flexibility, what you don't use, you lose – and quickly. The lesson: it is much better to stretch a little every day than to do a long stretching routine once or twice a week.

● **Hold a stretch on the tighter side of your body twice as long as on the more flexible side.** Prevent muscle imbalances by training the major muscle groups equally. If you are tighter on one side of your body, stretch that muscle for twice as long or repeat a stretch on that side to even things out.

● **Use proper body alignment.** It's easy to cheat when you stretch, but then you fail to get the stretch you need. The most typical 'cheating' is rounding your back. In 95 per cent of all stretches, you want to keep your spine long and flat. Before bending forward into any stretch, first inhale and extend upwards, creating as much space as you can between each vertebra in your spine. When you bend forward into a stretch, bend from the hips, not the waist. As you bend forward, your pubic bone should move forward while your tail bone (coccyx) moves back and up.

Compressed neck and spine

Extended neck and spine

Straight back

Rounded back

Bending at the waist

Bending at the hips

GOOD TECHNIQUE

POOR TECHNIQUE

● **Stretch after every walk, run, bike ride, aerobic class or any other cardiovascular activity.** Your muscles are at their most flexible and pliable after your workout, making your stretching more effective. After any activity designed to increase your heart rate, spend about 5 to 10 minutes cooling down and bringing your heart rate back to normal. Then do the full sequence of stretches outlined on page 135.

● **Hang.** Grab a pull-up bar and just hang from it – no pulling or swinging – for a minute or two. It's surprisingly refreshing and can do a lot of good for your spine, as well as your arm, shoulder and chest muscles. A great place to do it is on the climbing frame at a children's playground. However, if you haven't exercised for a while, or have a history of shoulder problems, ask your doctor first about this one, since you require your hands and shoulders to hold your entire body weight.

☆ **Dance your way to flexibility once a week in a dance class.** A Swedish study published in the *Journal of Strength Conditioning Research* tested 20 cross-country skiers for flexibility. Half the skiers took a dance class, and the other half served as a control group. Within three months, the skiers who took the weekly dance class improved the flexibility of their spines and consequently also increased their agility and ski speed on a slalom and hurdle test.

● **Stretch every time you get out of the car.** Even short periods of driving can cause back pain if you don't periodically stretch it out. When you get out of the car, lean backwards. Stand with your feet shoulder-width apart, put your hand in the small of your back and lean backwards using your hand to support your lower back. Then bend forward and place your hands on your knees. Exhale as you round your back and tuck in your chin. Then flatten your back, inhaling as you go. Hold each position for a count of two, repeating in both directions ten times.

● **Stretch your legs as you wait in a queue.** If you're stuck in a queue, stand on your toes, as high as you can, for as long as you can. Then, with your feet back on the ground, lift the toes of your right foot as high as they can go without lifting your heel, and hold for 20 seconds. Do the same with your left foot. These simple moves are good for any other occasion when you are on your feet for a long time.

● **Release your neck whenever you're on hold during a call.** Get a speakerphone or a headset. The next time someone puts you on hold, do some neck rolls or, if you're at home, get down on the floor and start doing your stretching routine.

☺ **Stretch during TV time.** Sprawl out on the floor and again go through your stretching routine, doing the three stretches described on page 135. If you feel good, do them a second and third time. If you do these stretches later in the day, your muscles will be warmed up from your daily activities. If nothing else, make a point of stretching during the commercials.

● **Rest your legs up a wall before going to bed every night.** Sit with one hip as close to the wall as you can get it. Then lie on your back and extend your legs up the wall, so that your bottom, the backs of your thighs and your heels touch the wall. You'll feel a mild stretch in your legs as gravity encourages fluids to drain out of your legs, back up to your heart. Hold the position for 5 minutes.

AFTERNOON routine

● **Near the end of your working day, do another 2 minute stretch routine.** Because your muscles are relatively warm and pliable from walking around all day, now is the perfect time to do the following static stretches. Some research suggests that flexibility peaks between 2.30pm and 4pm, due to the body's natural circadian rhythms. So although you'll achieve some benefit no matter what time of day you stretch, an afternoon routine may help you to gain more flexibility faster.

1 **LATERAL SIDE STRETCH**
Sit on the edge of your office chair with your feet on the floor. Place your left palm against the seat of the chair. Reach your right arm overhead. Extend upwards through your spine, then bend sideways to the left. Hold for 20 seconds, release, then repeat on the other side.

2 **HIP OPENER** Sit on a chair with your feet on the floor. Lift your right leg and place your right foot on your left thigh. Lean forward from the hips. Keep your back straight. Hold for 20 seconds, release, then repeat with your left leg.

3 **CHEST STRETCH** Stand with your feet under your hips. Clasp your hands behind your back. Roll your shoulders up, back, then down, feeling your chest open. Squeeze your shoulder blades together. To increase the stretch, lift your arms. Hold for 20 seconds and release.

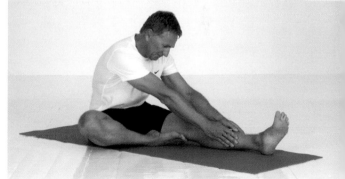

4 **SEATED HAMSTRING STRETCH** Sit on the floor with your left leg extended. Place your right foot against your left thigh. Lengthen your spine and bend forward from the hips. Don't let your back arch. Hold for 20 seconds. Repeat with your right leg extended.

WALKING

It's so simple and convenient it couldn't possibly count as exercise, right? Wrong. Study after study shows that regular moderate walking can help you to lose weight and reduce your risk of heart disease. In a study published in *Diabetes Research in Clinical Practice*, Japanese researchers tested obese men before and after they joined a one-year modest walking plan. All they did was increase the number of steps they took during their daily activities. The result: their blood pressure and cholesterol levels improved and the amount of body fat around their abdomen – the dangerous kind that leads to higher rates of heart disease and diabetes – significantly decreased. Here are some ways both to get more walking into your life and to reap the most benefits from every step.

29 WAYS TO DO IT BETTER AND MORE FREQUENTLY

☆**Learn the basics.** Before you take your next step outdoors, you need to know how much walking to do, and how often. Here are the facts:

● For it to be exercise, walk at a pace that has you breathing heavily, but still able to talk.

● Your goal, first and foremost, is to walk five days a week, 30 minutes a walk. Do that, and you are getting the base-level amount of exercise that research says should maintain your health and vigour.

● Don't assume you can reach that goal quickly. Walking hard for 30 minutes can be difficult at first. Walk for as long as feels comfortable during the first week, even if it's just to the postbox and back. Each subsequent week, increase that amount by no more than 10 per cent.

● Start every walk with 5 minutes of easy-paced walking, about the same pace at which you'd do your grocery shopping, to get your body warmed up. Then, cool down at the end of each walk with another 5 minutes of easy-paced walking. This allows your heart rate to speed up and slow down gradually.

● When you reach your target of 30 minutes a day, five days a week, set a new target. Either you should up your walking habit by increasing your time, or you might be ready for new forms of exercise, such as strength-building exercises twice a week.

● **Walk for entertainment one day a week.** Instead of walking around your local area, walk through a park, an art gallery or a shopping centre. First circle the perimeter of your location at your usual brisk pace. Then wander through again more slowly to take in the sights.

● **Walk with a friend.** If you have a friend expecting you, you're more likely to get out of bed on cold winter mornings

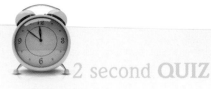

2 second QUIZ

Walk or run?
ANSWER: **WALK.**

Although runners and other high-energy athletes may scoff at walking, saying that it doesn't burn enough calories to result in real weight loss, research has shown time and time again that a regular walking programme, mile for mile, has just as beneficial an effect on your waistline. And as is clearly documented, people are far more likely to stick with a walking rather than a running regimen.

or skip the cafeteria for a lunchtime walk. If one of you backs out for any reason, put £1 in a kitty. If you manage to build up a substantial sum, donate it to charity.

● **Pick a charity and pledge to contribute a small sum for every mile that you walk.** You'll take pride in the fact that you are walking for something beyond yourself, which will motivate you to walk faster and for longer. After every walk, mark the amount you owe on a chart then, when you reach your target amount, send off a cheque.

☆**Use a pedometer.** These nifty gadgets measure how far you've walked in steps and miles or kilometres. They provide motivation by spurring you to meet a particular goal and showing you if you've met it. And research shows that they work. In one US study of 510 people, those who wore a pedometer automatically increased the amount of steps they took in a day. Often, pedometers hook onto your belt and are small and easy to use.

Walk your way to health with a pedometer.

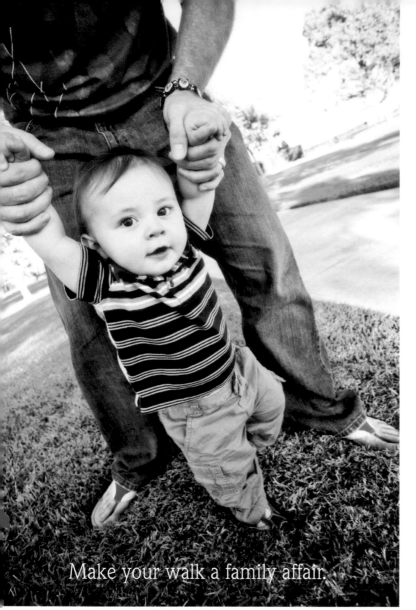

Make your walk a family affair.

active'. Using a pedometer, find your baseline of how many steps you normally take in a day. Then, increase that amount by at least 200 steps a day until you reach 10,000 to 12,500 daily steps.

● **Take the entire family on your daily walks.** Not only will you be exhibiting good fitness habits for your children, but you'll also be able to supervise them while you walk rather than getting a babysitter. If your children walk too slowly, ask them to ride their bikes or roller skate beside you. To keep everyone entertained, play your usual repertoire of long car-trip games such as I Spy. You can also try a treasure hunt, where you start out with a list of items to check off during your walk.

● **Improve your walking posture.** Proper posture will reduce discomfort as you walk and help you to burn more fat and calories. So when you go on your next walk, readjust yourself as follows:
• Stand tall with your spine elongated and breastbone lifted. This allows room for your lungs to expand fully.
• Keep your head straight with your eyes focused forward and shoulders relaxed. Avoid slumping your shoulders forward or hunching them towards your ears.
• Roll your feet from heel to toe. As you speed up, take smaller, more frequent steps. This protects your knees and gives your bottom a good workout.
• Allow your arms to swing freely.
• Firm your tummy and flatten your back as you walk to prevent lower back pain. Hold in your lower stomach around your waistband. Make sure you continue to breathe normally.

● **Once a week, complete your errands on foot.** If you live within a mile of your town centre or supermarket, start from

● **Aim for 10,000 steps a day.** Don't let that amount scare you. Most people walk about 5,500 to 7,500 steps during an average day as they amble to and from meetings, to the water cooler, to the postbox. In fact, researchers in the field consider 5,000 steps a day a 'sedentary lifestyle'. Studies have found that you should be able to cover 7,499 steps a day without participating in formal sports or exercise. If you reach 10,000 steps a day, you're considered 'active', while 12,500 steps a day earns you the title of 'highly

your house. If you live out in the middle of nowhere, drive to within a mile of your destination, park and walk the rest of the way there and back. You'll be surprised how much you can accomplish on foot and, even better, how many people you'll meet along the way.

● **Breathe deeply as you walk to a count of 1-2-3.** Many people unintentionally hold their breath when they exercise, then suddenly feel breathless and tired. Oxygen is invigorating, and muscles need it to create energy. So as you inhale, bring the air to the deepest part of your lungs by expanding your ribs outwards and your tummy forward and inhale for a count of three. Then exhale fully through your mouth, also to a count of three.

▐▐▐▶ **Periodically increase the pace.** Boredom can quickly bring a walk to a premature end. Keep your mind and your body engaged by increasing the pace or challenging yourself by trudging up a hill from time to time. Every 10 to 15 minutes, complete a 2 to 3 minute surge. During your surge, try to catch a real or imaginary walker ahead of you.

● **Take your dog with you (or get a dog).** Once your dog gets used to your walks, he or she will look forward to them and give you a gentle nudge (or annoying whine) on the days you try to get out of it. There's nothing more effective than a set of puppy-dog eyes to extract your bottom from the couch and get you out the door. In addition to walking locally, consider signing up for a dog agility class (try the Kennel Club, www.thekennelclub.org.uk, for more information). During the class, you and your dog will circumvent a course with see-saws, hurdles, tunnels and other obstacles. (Your dog tackles the obstacles.

You run or walk alongside and shout the appropriate command.) Both you and your dog will get a great workout and you'll end up with a better-behaved and calmer dog as a result. If you don't have a dog, offer to walk a neighbour's dog twice a week. The commitment will keep you motivated.

● **Explore on your walks.** You can walk anywhere at any time, from your neighbourhood to your local shops to a local nature trail. You can even walk laps around your office building. But rather than walking the same old tired route day in and day out, use your walks as a way to experience and explore the great outdoors. Varying your route and terrain will do more than keep you mentally engaged. It will also help you to target different leg muscles.

simple as taking a 5 minute walk break around the building after completing a big project at work. Such short walking breaks will refresh your mind, so you can return to work with more vigour. In fact, research shows that most people can focus at top capacity for only 30 minutes at a time. After that, concentration begins to drop off. So your intermittent walk breaks may actually make you more productive.

● **Walk and talk.** Use a cordless phone and walk around the house or up and down the stairs as you chat with friends or conduct your business. This is a also a good way to make use of those long times spent on hold. You get some heart-healthy exercise, and the exercise will help you to maintain your mental cool. Use your pedometer to count your steps and you'll get the added bonus of feeling as if you have accomplished something rather than wasting time.

● **Apply some Vaseline.** If you're a long-distance walker or somewhat overweight, chafing clothes can make you want to call it quits. You can solve the problem by wearing skin-hugging

Avoid chafing with Vaseline.

clothing and applying Vaseline to your sensitive areas. The Vaseline acts like a barrier to protect your skin.

● **Walk faster earlier in your walk.** If you want to increase the amount of fat you burn, add some bursts of faster walking near the beginning of your walk, rather than going for a final spurt. A study in the *European Journal of Applied Physiology* found that people exercising burned more fat and felt less tired when they inserted their faster segments towards the beginning of a workout. You'll speed up your heart rate early and keep it elevated for the rest of your walk.

● **Take light weights (1kg to 2kg) on your walks.** Periodically work in arm exercises as you walk. This does more than increase the benefit of the workout. Carrying weights also builds muscle, and each pound of muscle burns about 30 to 50kcal more a day. Build a couple of pounds of muscle in your arms alone and you'll burn an extra 100kcal a day – even while you're channel surfing. Or try isometric exercises of the arms, chest and abdominal muscles. For instance, as you walk, go through the action of throwing a punch in slow motion. As you extend your arm, tense the muscles along it and do the same as you retract it. You should feel tension in your triceps, biceps, deltoids and pectoral muscles. Then repeat with your arms going straight up and down, or out to the side. You can also tense your chest muscles by bringing your hands together in front of your body and contracting across the chest and shoulders. Do this rhythmically to match your gait. Also try doing curls with no weights. Simply curl your arms alternately, in rhythm with your gait. Each time you curl your forearms, tense your biceps.

WEEKENDS

If you were to believe some of the adverts on television, you'd think that most of us spend our weekends cycling, rock climbing, playing games on the beach and generally being active. A look at the shopping centre car park on a Saturday afternoon paints a different picture. The weekend has become a time of errands, shopping and finishing up the work we didn't get to during the week. For too many of us, our spirit of adventure is being satisfied by the thought of finding a great bargain. And for parents, any thrill-seeking is being fulfilled through our children, as we shuttle them to and from parties and classes, watching from the sidelines. It's time to reclaim your weekends – or at least, a good-sized chunk of them. Here are suggestions for squeezing in some life-affirming weekend activity.

20 IDEAS FOR MORE ACTIVE DAYS OFF

Be one of the children.

walking, cycling, birdwatching or running clubs in most areas that have regular weekend events. Fitness centres and regional parks are a great place to start your search for the right one for you.

▶ **Be one of the children.** Don't just push them out the door and spend the afternoon inside reading or cleaning. Join them. Find a tree and climb it with them. Spend the day skating or cycling or playing tag. After all, even those of us with ageing bodies have some childishness still inside us, just aching to get out. See page 154, 'Family Fun', for more ways to stay fit with your family.

● **Take the family camping.** There's nothing quite like the great outdoors to put your body in a calorie-burning state, or to create happy, memorable times for your children. After you've set up your site, you can look into other activities such as swimming, canoeing and hiking.

● **Make a list of weekend fitness activities and choose one activity from the list every week.** The more varied your weekend fitness routine, the more likely you'll be to stay active at the weekends. On your list, you might write hiking, canoeing, walking, cycling, birdwatching and other activities.

● **Keep a fitness kit in your car.** Stock your car with a bat and ball, football, Frisbee or other favourite fitness items. Be sure to include a pair of trainers. You never know when you'll find yourself away from home with a little free time. If your fitness kit is stocked and ready, you'll have everything you need for fun.

● **Train for a race.** Whether you walk, run, cycle or do some other sport, signing up for a race will give you the incentive to train at the weekends. Suddenly fitness becomes the top priority in your life. Plus, this is what serious athletes do – complete their longer workout sessions at the weekends, when they have time away from work.

● **Take calisthenics breaks.** If you find yourself working at the office (or at home) over the weekend, take a 10 minute break every hour and do star jumps, lunges, push-ups and crunches. Over the course of the day, you'll have exercised for more than 60 minutes.

● **Combine physically active work with pure indulgence.** For instance, chop some logs or gather firewood as the physically active part of your day, then sit in front of the fire with someone special for the pure indulgence part. Or clean up your garden by day, then have a barbecue that evening. Or take a long walk, knowing you have a well-stocked picnic basket waiting for you in the car.

HOLIDAYS

When we take a holiday, what many of us want most is simply to relax. And so we spend long, lazy days on a deckchair and socialise the night away drinking and indulging in calorific desserts. Too often, we return home flabbier than we've been since, well, our last holiday. It doesn't have to be this way. Active holidays can often be the most relaxing of all. Yes, really. It's all about defining what an active holiday is. The idea is to try to spend 2 to 4 hours a day doing things. Walking the city streets. Exploring a nature reserve. Going to a zoo. These kinds of activities improve your physical and mental health and make holidays memorable. Here are some fresh ideas to make your trips away as pleasurable as they are active and healthy.

13 TIPS FOR ACTIVELY INDULGENT TRAVEL

Family FUN

If you have children living at home, this chapter is for you. It's also for grandparents, and for all the uncles and aunts who love to spend time with their nieces and nephews, and all of the babysitters, day-care and after-school workers, neighbours and school volunteers. In short, it's for any adult who spends time with children. The message of this chapter is twofold: first, that you have a wonderful opportunity to get some fun, high-quality exercise by playing with children; second, that you have a responsibility to teach them about the joys and importance of exercise. Engaging your children in a health-promoting lifestyle should be a priority for every loving parent. But if you want trim and healthy kids, you have to get trim and healthy yourself. This is how to do it.

39 WAYS TO USE THE ULTIMATE EXERCISE MACHINES – CHILDREN

● **Go on a treasure hunt.** Here's a great way to keep the family fit and teach your children about trust, teamwork and problem solving at the same time. Take them to a local park and set an expedition course on a map, circling various 'checkpoints'. Take turns navigating to each point on the map and leading the team to each destination. 'Start out with an easy course in an open park, then progress to a trail system,' suggests Claire Small, a musculoskeletal physiotherapist with London's Pure Sports Medicine. 'Stay together and explore terrain features, study map clues, and look for the secret treasure.' Sound too complicated? Then merely go hunting for insects, animals or flowers. You can't entertain a young child much better than finding a slumbering beetle under a log or rock.

☆ **Plan 10 minute spurts of activity followed by 5 minute rest periods.** Don't force your adult exercise programme on your children. That's a recipe for disaster. Studies published in the journal *Medicine & Science in Sports & Exercise* show that forcing children to participate in structured exercise turns them off exercise later in life. Instead, take advantage of their natural tendency to participate in intermittent and sporadic play and exercise bouts. A game of tag is a perfect example. Children's bodies are designed to sprint and rest, sprint and rest. Because they are easily distracted and incapable of long periods of focused activity, they will resist long exercise sessions that don't include rest periods.

● **Hold a sports party.** Rather than the typical tea, cakes and pass-the-parcel birthday party, hold your child's birthday party in an active location, such as a roller skating or ice-skating rink, a ski or climbing centre, or an indoor 'soft

A SERIOUS message

Childhood obesity experts in the UK discovered that more than 2.3 million children in this country are overweight or obese. Not only that, many under-12s already show signs of high blood pressure, high cholesterol and liver disease. These statistics have serious implications:
● Children are now subject to an epidemic of Type 2 diabetes, a disease that once occurred exclusively at or beyond middle age in adults.
● The obesity epidemic holds more harm for today's children than exposure to tobacco, drugs and alcohol combined.
● If they don't mend their ways, today's children may well have a shorter life expectancy than their parents, as they eat themselves into an early grave.

Studies show that the family environment is one of the strongest predictors of childhood obesity. In one study, children of sedentary parents (so-called couch potatoes) were more likely to gain weight and become overweight than the children of active parents.

One important fact for parents and carers to remember: you and your child burn more calories standing than sitting, walking than standing. The more you move, the more you burn. And it doesn't really matter what type of activity you choose: if you are moving and having fun, you're burning calories and getting in shape. It's that simple.

play' area. You don't have to limit this to parties. A growing number of indoor playgrounds offer structured games every week. Or you can have your own 'no particular reason' party. Children might not think of what they're doing as exercise – but it is.

● **Play 'chase my shadow'.** The children have to jump and run to catch your shadow, then vice versa.

● **Play follow-the-leader with one or more children.** Line up in single file and weave your way through the house or garden. Every few steps, hop, skip, jump or do some other movement that your followers must imitate. Once the children

ARM strength

More than 70 years ago, you rarely heard of people lifting weights to keep their arms strong. They didn't have to. Washing clothes by hand, scrubbing pots, chopping wood and scrubbing floors all maintained the muscle mass we needed to stay strong as we aged. Today, of course, things have changed. Modern conveniences mean we rarely call upon our arm muscles to do much of anything. Over a lifetime, this can cause your muscles to wither away. You get weaker and weaker, daily tasks become harder and your body puts on weight and grows more susceptible to disease as you become more and more sedentary. So don't think of strengthening your arms as an act of vanity. The tips in this chapter will help you to fit some arm-strengthening moves into your routines.

17 WAYS TO EXERCISE WITH – OR WITHOUT – WEIGHTS

● **Each autumn, plant bulbs on three consecutive weekends.** Make each planting session last at least an hour. Congratulations – that's your arm workout for the week. Digging in your garden will strengthen your hands, wrists, forearms, upper arms and shoulders. Your hard work will pay off in the spring, when your daffodils and tulips bloom.

● **Stop using weedkiller on your garden.** Yes, this will encourage weeds to grow with wild abandon (even with mulch). That's good, because your job is to get down on your hands and knees once a week to rip weeds out of the ground. Leaning onto your hands as you weed will build arm, shoulder and upper back strength, and yanking the weeds provides an extra dose of arm-building strength. Just remember to alternate hands as you reach and pull so that you work both arms equally.

▶ **Cut your own wood.** If you have a real fire, the chances are you're burning pre-cut logs. If you have the option, though, go out and chop your own wood. Do 30 minutes of log chopping every weekend. Too much at once and it's bad for your back. But in small doses, cutting wood is amazingly good exercise.

● **Scrub the floors on your hands and knees once a week.** Not only will you have cleaner floors than a mop provides, but you'll strengthen your arms at the same time.

● **Bake bread once a week.** You'll strengthen your arms, shoulders and hands as you simultaneously soothe away stress. There's little more calming than the repetitive motion of kneading dough and nothing more pleasing than the smell of bread in the oven. Plus, home-baked

bread – kneaded with your own two hands – tastes better than anything from the shops or made in the breadmaker.

● **Make your own pizza dough and pastry instead of buying them pre-made.** The forward and back action of using a rolling pin is a great arm and shoulder workout. And your family will thank you for your effort later, as no shop-bought product compares to homemade.

In PERSPECTIVE

Build strength

When people in their 20s are described as 'strong', chances are the subject is muscles. Call someone in his or her 60s 'strong', and you're probably talking about character. It's time to change that perception.

The benefits of strong muscles – particularly for people above 50, especially women – are vast. Steve Nance, Performance Director at Pure Sports Medicine and Leeds Rugby Union Club says it's also very good for women to do strength training to prevent osteoporosis. Here's why building stronger muscles is one of the best health-boosting pursuits:

● Strong muscles help you to lose weight. Muscle tissue burns as much as 15 times more calories per day than fat tissue does – even when at rest.

● Strong muscles are healthy for your heart. That's because they can perform better with less oxygen, meaning the heart doesn't have to pump too hard when you are active. By extension, strong muscles are good for your blood pressure.

● Strong muscles protect your joints and your back. More muscle power means you put less strain on your joints and connective tissue when lifting or exerting yourself. And that's important both for treating and preventing arthritis.

● Strong muscles improve your looks and give you a mental boost. You feel more energised, and prouder about yourself.

● Strong muscles require active living. You can't get strong muscles from a pill, a meal or a herb. The mere fact that you have strong muscles means you're being active.

● Strong muscles help to fight free radicals (see page 91). Research shows that when people lift weights regularly, they suffer less damage from free radicals than those who are sedentary.

ARM EXERCISES for TV ad-breaks

⭐ **Do each of the following exercises at least once a week.** For even better effect, do them twice a week. An easy system: do one exercise each night during a 3 minute commercial break on television (have a rest day on Sunday). Do three slow sets of 10 to 12 repetitions, with 20 seconds of breathing time between sets. This will require keeping a set of dumbbells next to the couch. Beginners should use 2kg dumbbells, and more active adults should try 5kg or 7kg versions. These simple exercises are suggested by Steve Nance, Performance Director at Pure Sports Medicine and Leeds Rugby Union Club.

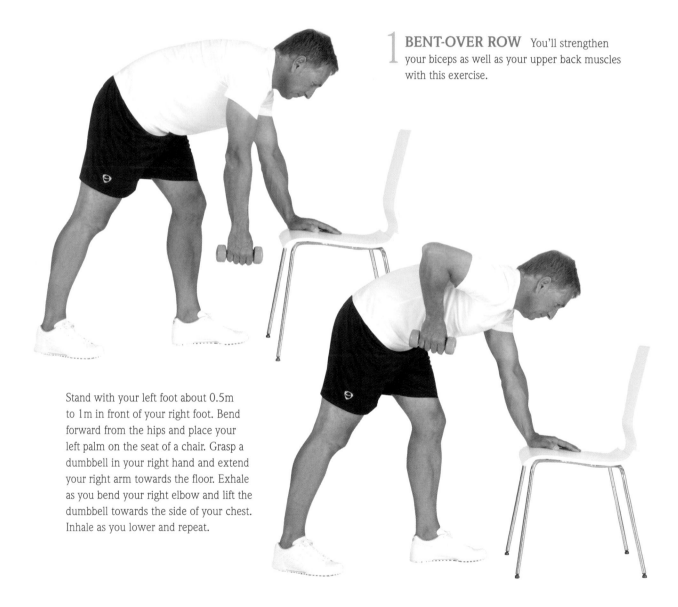

1 **BENT-OVER ROW** You'll strengthen your biceps as well as your upper back muscles with this exercise.

Stand with your left foot about 0.5m to 1m in front of your right foot. Bend forward from the hips and place your left palm on the seat of a chair. Grasp a dumbbell in your right hand and extend your right arm towards the floor. Exhale as you bend your right elbow and lift the dumbbell towards the side of your chest. Inhale as you lower and repeat.

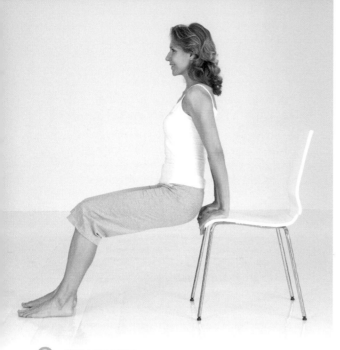
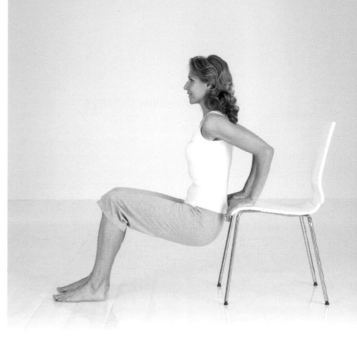

2 CHAIR DIP

This exercise, above, strengthens your triceps, the muscles along the back of your upper arms (the ones that flap about when you wave goodbye) and your chest muscles.

Sit on the edge of a sturdy chair. Place your palms on the seat of the chair, at either side of your bottom, with your fingers facing forward. Place your feet flat on the floor with your knees bent. Press into your hands and lift your bottom about an inch up and forward, until you can clear the seat of the chair. Inhale as you bend your elbows, lowering your bottom towards the floor. Keeping your elbows close to your sides, exhale as you extend your arms and return to the starting position. Be careful you're not cheating by pushing yourself back up with your legs rather than your arms.

As you gain strength, you can increase the challenge by extending your legs and placing only your heels on the floor.

3 BICEPS CURL

This exercise, right, strengthens your biceps, the muscles along the front of your upper arms.

Grasp a dumbbell in each hand. Extend your arms at your sides with your palms facing forward. Exhale as you curl your hands towards your shoulders, keeping your elbows close to your sides. Inhale as you lower the weights. .

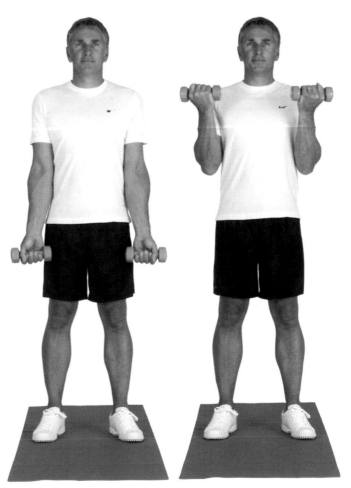

2 second QUIZ

Fast lifting or slow lifting?
ANSWER: **SLOW LIFTING.**

The research is clear: the slower you move the weight, the better. In one American study involving 147 people, participants who lifted slowly – taking a full 14 seconds to complete one repetition – gained more strength than participants who spent just 7 seconds on each repetition. Plus, even though the slow weightlifting group completed fewer repetitions of each exercise (just 4 to 6 compared to the faster group's 8 to 12), they still gained more strength. Slower lifting may help to increase strength because it prevents you from using momentum or cheating with improper technique.

● **Trade in your electric mixer for a whisk and wooden spoon.** You'll build arm strength as you use your own elbow grease to mix batter. Be sure to use both hands to work your arms evenly.

● **Make an omelette rather than fried eggs.** Fill it with at least three different vegetables, such as spinach, mushrooms and onions. You'll not only use your arms to whisk the eggs and chop the veggies, but you'll also improve your health by incorporating veg into your morning meal.

☺ **Use a cast-iron pot for most of your cooking** – and store it in the drawer under the cooker. That way, you need to lift the heavy pot onto the hob each time you need it – building more arm strength with every meal.

☺ **Have a large cleaver for everyday chopping and cooking.** Professional chefs love cleavers for their weight and super-sharp, slightly rounded edge. Use one too and you'll give your hand and arm a great workout while you cook.

● **Pour water out of a large jug.** The weight of a large jug may do wonders for your arms (4 litres of water weighs more than 3.5kg). Curl your jug five times – by bending your elbow and bringing your hand to your shoulder – before pouring.

● **Spend 10 minutes every working day building up resistance in your office.** You have everything you need in the office to keep your arms in great shape. Here are some great office-based arm exercises:
● Desk curl. Place your palms against the underside of your desk with your elbows bent. Push up into the desk with your palms, as if you were trying to lift the desk off the floor. Hold for a count of five, release, then repeat until you feel the burn. This strengthens your biceps.
● Desk push. Place your palms against the top of your desk with your elbows bent. Press into the desktop with all your might. Hold for a count of five, release, then repeat until you feel the burn. This strengthens your triceps.
● Desk push-up. Stand about 0.5m away from your desk. Keep your feet in place and lean forward from your ankles, placing your palms on top of the desk. Your body should form a straight line from your ankles to your head. Bend your elbows as you lower your chest towards the desk. Straighten your elbows as you push away. Keep your elbows in close to your sides the entire time. This works your triceps.

● **Eat a steak on the nights you work out.** Researchers at the University of Wollongong in New South Wales, Australia, put 28 participants aged 60-plus on one of two diet and exercise programmes. Both programmes contained weightlifting exercises and a diet that included 20 per cent protein. One diet, however, included 700g of red meat a week (the amount in three medium steaks), whereas the other included just over 350g of red meat (the amount in 1½ medium steaks). After 12 weeks, those with the extra red meat increased their muscle strength more than those who ate less red meat. Researchers suspect the extra red meat supplies additional amino acids needed for muscle growth. If you plan to increase your consumption of red meat, choose lean cuts, such as sirloin, rather than rib-eye. That helps to protect your heart as you build up your strength.

● **Hang your laundry outside instead of using the tumble-dryer.** As well as saving money on your electric bill, you'll get in a mild arm workout. As you carry the laundry basket to the clothes line, curl it up and down, bringing your hands to your shoulders. You can also hold it overhead, bending, then extending your elbows.

● **Curl your shopping.** When you arrive home from the supermarket, carry one bag in each hand. As you walk from the car to the kitchen, curl your groceries by lifting your hands towards your shoulders, keeping your elbows close to your sides. By the time you bring in all of the bags of shopping, you'll have given your biceps a good workout – and you'll have burned some extra calories by making the extra trips to and from the car.

☆ **Try these isometric exercises.** These types of exercise are performed against something that doesn't move, like a wall. By pushing against the immovable object, tension builds up in your muscles, increasing their strength. Hold each for 5 to 8 seconds, and repeat five to ten times.
● Press your hands together as hard as you can ten times for 5 seconds at a time. This will really make a difference to your arm strength after a couple of weeks. Try it every time you sit down to watch TV.
● Stand with your legs apart about 30cm from the wall and push against the wall as if you were trying to move it.
● Stand in the doorway with your legs straight and knees locked. Press your hands upwards against the top of the door frame, holding for several seconds, then relaxing. Repeat at least ten times.
● Extend both arms to the side of the doorway with your palms shoulder high, facing outwards. With both arms, press hard against the sides of the door frame. Hold for several seconds, relax, then repeat up to ten times.
● Extend both arms to the sides of the doorway, arms down, palms facing in. With the back of your hands, press hard against the sides of the frame. Hold for a few seconds, relax, then repeat up to ten times.

Peg up your washing for a swift arm workout.

Reminder

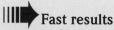 **Fast results**
These are tips that deliver benefits particularly quickly – in some cases, immediately.

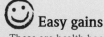 **Easy gains**
These are health boosters that offer the best value for the least amount of effort.

☆ **Super-effective**
This is advice that scientific research or widespread usage by experts has shown to be especially effective.

ABS & BACK
strength

Your abs (abdominal muscles) and back are the core of your body, the power centre from which all movement originates. Strengthen them and you'll move with more power and grace. Strong abdominal muscles also help to support and move your spine, protecting your back from injury. Finally, strengthen the lowest part of your core – your pelvic-floor muscles – and you'll prevent incontinence and may even improve your sex life. In this chapter, you'll discover a whole new world of opportunities for abdominal and back strengthening beyond the basic crunch.

17 WAYS TO FEEL LESS CRUNCHED DURING YOUR ROUTINE

● **If you walk for fitness, squeeze your bottom.** As you walk, imagine someone is poking you in the bottom with a sharp instrument. Tighten your bottom muscles but don't squeeze them together. As you firm and lift your bottom muscles, you'll strengthen them. You can also work your abs as you walk by imagining you have a zip along the midline of your abdomen. Picture yourself zipping up a tight pair of jeans. As you pull the zip up your abdomen, feel your torso lengthen and your abdomen firm up. Keep your abs zipped up and your bottom tucked under throughout your walks and you'll strengthen your core even as you burn fat.

● **While driving, tighten your tummy and pelvic-floor muscles.** Starting with your pubic area, begin to tighten from the bottom up. Once you squeeze your pelvic floor, suck in your lower belly and then upper belly towards your spine as you exhale. Hold for a count of five, then release and repeat 10 to 20 times.

● **When you're nervous,** tighten and release your abdominal muscles over and over again. You'll strengthen your abs and take your mind off your anxiety. This is a particularly good exercise for when you are nervous about an upcoming speech or presentation.

● **During commercial breaks on TV,** sit on the edge of your chair and lift your feet off the floor, bringing your knees into your chest. Lower and repeat 10 to 15 times.

● **Whenever you find yourself standing in a queue,** lift one foot off the floor and try to hold your balance. You'll feel the myriad muscles in your abdomen and back firing up to help to steady your body. Be sure to alternate your feet.

In PERSPECTIVE

Achieving flat abs

So what does it take to have an abdomen that is so strong, so slender, that it reveals beautifully symmetric, perfectly arranged muscles? There are a few surprises in the answers.

Most of all, it takes being very, very lean. For most people, much of their fat lies in the abdomen, and much of that abdominal fat lies between the skin and abdominal muscles. That layer of fat covers up the shapeliness of the muscles. So models and athletes with 'six-pack abs' must have very low body fat to reveal that musculature. Sit-ups didn't get them that way – you cannot 'spot reduce' fat from your belly using abs exercises. To melt the fat off your body, it requires a low-calorie diet and lots of aerobic exercise such as cycling, walking or running.

Of course, it does take targeted exercise to create big, shapely abdominal muscles. A lot, in fact. While most of us think of the abs as a simple band of muscles across the top of the abdomen, there are many separate abdominal muscles, with names such as 'obliques' and 'transversus abdominis'. People serious about their abs know all these muscles, and target each one for exercise. A thorough abs workout could involve ten different abdominal exercises.

Is all this necessary? Maybe for models, but not for you. What's important is that your ab muscles are conditioned well enough to support your back and allow you to twist, turn and lift without a challenge. If you are at a healthy weight but have a little fat covering your abdominal muscles, consider yourself well ahead of the game.

☺ **Do abdominal exercises as a warm-up for your workout.** The typical workout starts out with 5 or 10 minutes of walking or marching to get your body warmed up and your blood flowing. In truth, that can be boring. Instead, do your abdominal work. Because your abdomen consists of large muscle groups, abdominal work is very warming for the body. Just 5 to 10 minutes of abdominal exercises will warm you up just as well as walking, and give you some good muscle building at the same time.

ABS & BACK ball exercises

● **Use your exercise ball to do abs and back exercises.** Whenever you perform abdominal-strengthening movements on a ball, you use more of your core muscles for every movement. Try the traditional crunch on the ball, shown on page 174, along with these additional ball moves, courtesy of Claire Small, a specialist musculoskeletal physiotherapist and co-founder/director of London-based Pure Sports Medicine.

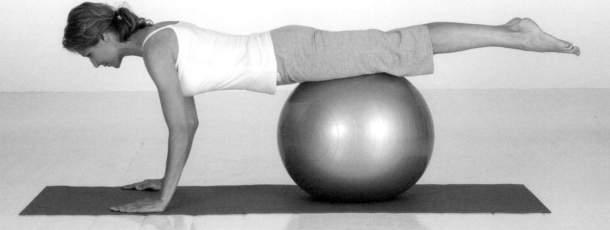

1 **KNEE FOLD-UP** Start in a push-up position with your thighs or shins on the ball and your palms on the floor under your chest. Exhale as you bend your knees and bring your shins and ball in towards your chest. Inhale as you straighten your legs. Repeat 10 to 15 times.

2 **KNEELING PUSH-OUTS**   Kneel on the floor with the ball in front of you, keeping your head in a neutral position, with your chin tucked in and your spine stable. Clasp your hands and press the bottoms of your hands into the ball. Lift your feet and shins and balance on your knees. Exhale as you press your hands into the ball and roll the ball forward. Your knees will stay in place, but your feet and shins will rise and your torso will lean forward. Raise yourself back up and repeat 15 times.

3 **ARM SWING**   Lie with your upper back on the ball, your knees bent and your feet on the floor. Clasp your hands together and extend your arms towards the ceiling, so that they are perpendicular with your torso.

Exhale and roll your torso to the left, lifting your right shoulder off the ball. Return to the starting position and repeat to the right, alternating sides. Complete 10 to 15 rolls on each side.

The most effective
ABDOMINAL EXERCISES

Researchers at San Diego State University have tested numerous abdominal exercises for their effectiveness; surprisingly, the quintessential crunch ranked only 11th out of the 13 exercises tested. Here are five of the best.

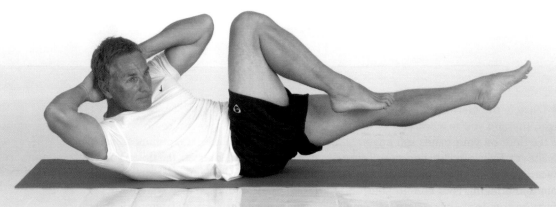

1 BICYCLE Lie on your back. Tuck in your tail bone (coccyx) and press your lower back against the floor. Place your fingertips behind your head and your elbows out to the sides. Bend your knees and lift your feet off the floor, keeping a 45 degree bend in your knees. Begin to pedal your legs, bringing your opposite elbow to the opposite knee as you extend your free leg.

2 BALL CRUNCH A large, air-filled exercise ball will wiggle under your back, causing you to recruit more muscles as you crunch.

Sit on the ball with your feet on the floor. Walk your feet away from the ball as you recline onto it. The ball should rest against your lower back and the top of your bottom. Your upper back and shoulders should not rest on the ball. With your fingertips behind your head, open your elbows to the sides. Tuck in your tail bone and exhale as you lift your shoulders. Lower and repeat.

3 CAPTAIN'S (ROMAN) CHAIR

Here's a simple way to adapt a gym exercise for home use. Most gyms have an ab-strengthening device where you sit with your forearms on padding, grip handholds and, while pressing your lower back against the back pad, you lift your legs off the floor, drawing your knees up towards your chest.

You can do this at home in a sturdy, armless chair. Sit up straight, grabbing the chair's edges just in front of your hips. Don't let your back arch or move – to protect your back and ensure you work your abs effectively. Supporting yourself with your hands, slowly draw your knees up towards your chest, keeping your lower back against the chair. Hold, slowly lower, then repeat.

4 EXTENDED LEG CRUNCH

Lie on your back. Extend your legs towards the ceiling and cross one ankle over the other. Place your fingertips behind your head with your elbows open to the sides. Tuck in your tail bone. Slowly lift your shoulders off the floor as you exhale. Lower and repeat.

5 REVERSE CRUNCH

Lie on your back. Bend your knees and lift your feet off the floor, forming a 90 degree angle between your thighs and calves. Place your fingertips behind your head with your elbows open to the sides. Cross your ankles. Press your lower back into the floor, tuck in your tail bone, and reach your shins towards the ceiling. For this exercise to be effective, it must be your pelvis that moves, not your hips (as in a tilt). Lower and repeat.

AB-STRENGTHENING ball routine

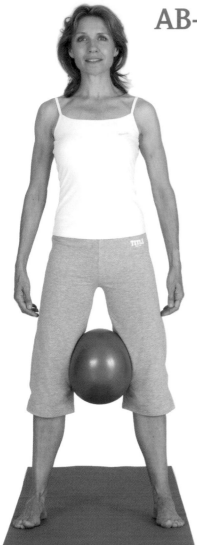

● **Use a children's ball as an abdominal strengthening aid.** Children's play balls or small (about 20cm), light fitness balls make great workout aids. To start, use one in the kitchen while cooking. Place the ball between your thighs, just above your knees. As you work, squeeze your inner thighs to hold the ball in place. This action fires up your pelvic floor and lower abdominal muscles. You can also use a small ball to increase the effectiveness of traditional abdominal exercises. Here are a few to try:

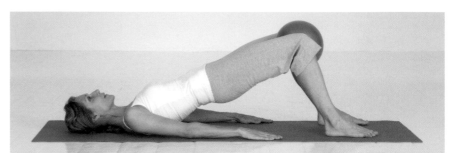

2 THE BRIDGE This exercise works your lower abdominal area, lower back and bottom. Lie on your back with your knees bent, feet on the floor and the ball between your thighs. Rest your arms at your sides with your palms down. Tuck in your tail bone (coccyx) and lift your hips and lower back off the floor. Lift only as high as you can while still keeping your tail bone tucked in. Hold for 10 to 20 seconds. Lower and repeat once or twice.

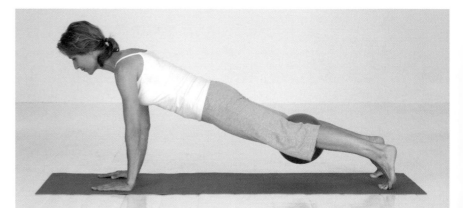

1 THE MOUNTAIN This exercise stretches your calves, helps your posture and, by adding in the small exercise ball, it works your lower abdominals as well.

Stand tall with the ball between your thighs. Lift your arches and squeeze the ball. Hold for 10 to 20 seconds. Release the ball, walk around a bit, then repeat the exercise once or twice.

3 THE PLANK This simple exercise challenges several body areas, including the shoulders, backs and abs. The small exercise ball brings even more pelvic muscles into the mix.

With the ball between your knees or thighs, come into a push-up position with your hands under your chest. Reach back through your heels and forward through the top of your head. Tuck in your tail bone. Hold for 10 to 20 seconds. Repeat once or twice.

LEG strength

Your legs contain perhaps the easiest muscles in your body to keep in shape. After all, they support the weight of your body and you use them every time you walk. Just being on the go can help you to tone and fine-tune them, and they, in turn, will help you to burn calories and keep the rest of your body fit. Add some leg-strengthening exercises, and you'll gain even more benefits without a lot of effort. A stronger pair of legs will help you to accomplish more every day. You'll climb stairs more easily and be able to bend your knees and squat down to pick up heavy objects, protecting your lower back from strain. To strengthen your legs and avoid injury, you must work all of the muscles in your legs equally. The following tips will incorporate thorough leg work seamlessly into your day.

19 WAYS TO FIRM UP YOUR HIPS, THIGHS AND BOTTOM

● **Whenever you stop at traffic lights,** tighten your thighs and bottom, over and over again. You will firm your leg muscles, boost blood flow (thus preventing the pins-and-needles sensation that tends to attack your bottom when you've been sitting in a car seat for too long) and give yourself something to focus on.

● **Before you get out of bed in the morning, do the clam.** Lie on your back, bring your feet together, and open your knees out to the sides. Then, as you exhale, lift your knees, bringing them together. Lower and repeat this exercise 10 to 15 times and you'll strengthen your inner thighs.

● **Do leg lifts as you cook dinner.** Flex your foot and lift your leg out to the side, lower it, then repeat 10 to 15 times. Make sure you move only at the hip – don't let your waist move. Then swap legs. You'll finish your leg workout before dinner time.

Healthy **INVESTMENT**

Ankle weights
One set of ankle weights allows you to do just about any leg exercise at home and you'll never have to set foot in the gym again to maintain shapely legs. In addition to the traditional leg lifts, you can use ankle weights to do other popular leg exercises such as hamstring curls and leg extensions, often performed on a machine at the gym. Look for ankle weights that allow you to add weight as you get stronger, and with Velcro straps rather than shoelaces for easy access and removal. Many of these weights contain small pockets into which you can insert or remove weighted bags. Try on the weights in the shop to make sure they feel comfortable.

● **If you walk for fitness, switch to a softer surface.** Your legs get a better workout when you walk on footpaths or sand rather than pavement. And softer surfaces transfer less impact to your joints, preventing strain to your knees and back.

☺ **Get up, place your palms against your desk** and do a series of donkey kicks when you find yourself falling asleep at your keyboard. Bend one knee, flex that foot and kick your leg back, as if you were a donkey kicking someone behind you. Alternate legs for 15 kicks in total. Then return to work refreshed and with a stronger bottom.

● **Instead of straining and reaching to get something** off a high shelf, step up on a stool. You'll strengthen your legs and protect your back.

● **Next time you find yourself at a wedding or other function** with a dance floor, do the twist. Or, do it in your living room tonight. Bend your knees and squat down as far as you comfortably can as you shimmy from side to side. You'll burn calories, have a few laughs and strengthen your legs – all at the same time.

● **Do the 'lunge walk' in the garden.** Your neighbours might laugh if they see you, but you'll have the last laugh when, in just minutes each day, you sculpt a toned pair of legs. During each step forward, bend your knees and sink down until both legs form 90 degree angles. Then press into your front heel to rise. Lift your back leg and knee all the way into your chest before planting it in front of you for the next lunge. This takes a little practice (see also page 182), but if you 'lunge walk' for 20 or 30 steps a day, your legs will be far stronger and shapelier.

THE SQUAT: king of the leg exercises

Can you do only one leg exercise and still see results? Yes, if that exercise is a squat. You can strengthen all of the muscles in your legs and bottom with either full squats or quarter-squats, says Steve Nance, Performance Director at Pure Sports Medicine in London and Leeds Rugby Union Club.

1 **FULL SQUAT** Stand with your feet slightly wider than hip distance apart. Tuck in your tail bone (coccyx), flatten your back and firm up your abdominal muscles. Inhale and slowly bend your knees as you sit back, as if you were going to sit back into a chair. Your upper body will lean slightly forward, but don't allow your lower back to arch or your spine to round. Bend your knees until your thighs are parallel with the floor. Then exhale as you press up through your heels and extend your legs in a fast, explosive motion. Repeat 10 to 15 times. Do this two or three times a week.

If you lack the leg strength to do a full squat or – more importantly – if you feel pain in your knees or back, try one of two variations.

Variation 1. Hold on to a doorknob with both hands as you squat. This removes some of your body weight from your legs and helps to keep your torso upright.

Variation 2. Squat with your back against a wall and a small 20cm diameter ball between your thighs. The ball keeps your thighs and knees in proper alignment, and the wall provides more support for your back.

2 **QUARTER-SQUAT** For this exercise, you'll do the same motion and use the same technique as the full squat, but you won't bend your knees quite so far. Rather than lowering your thighs to parallel, bend your knees only a quarter of the distance of the full squat before rising to the starting position. Repeat 10 to 15 times, two or three times a week.

KICKBOXING

● **Practise kickboxing moves** for 5 minutes every morning before putting on your trousers or skirt. There's nothing like seeing your bare thighs in the mirror to motivate you to do your kicks. Kick in all directions, mixing in front kicks, roundhouse kicks, side kicks and back kicks. No matter what kick you do, never fully extend your knee. This protects your knee joint.

1 **FRONT KICK** Pretend an opponent is standing in front of you and you wish to kick him or her in the groin (or in the stomach). Lift one knee into your chest, then forcefully extend your leg, smacking the top of your foot into your imaginary target. Recoil your leg quickly and follow up with the other leg in quick succession.

2 **ROUNDHOUSE KICK**
Pretend your opponent is standing in front of you and slightly to your left. Place your hands in a boxer's stance for balance. Bring your left knee diagonally into your chest. Snap your leg forward as you extend your foot and shin into your opponent's imaginary abdomen. Recoil quickly and follow up with 10 to 20 more kicks before switching sides.

3 **SIDE KICK** Pretend an opponent is standing to your left side. Place your hands in a boxer's stance for balance. Bend your left knee and bring your left foot towards your right knee. Then thrust it sideways to the left, into your opponent's imaginary abdomen. Do 10 to 20 on one side, then swap sides.

4 **BACK KICK** Pretend your opponent is standing behind you. Place your hands in a boxer's stance and turn your head and shoulders to look at your 'attacker'. Bring one leg in towards your chest, then thrust it behind you, trying to thrust your foot into your attacker's imaginary abdomen. Alternate with your other leg in rapid succession.

● **Mount the stairs two or three at a time.** This strengthens the gluteal muscles in your bottom and revs up your heart rate, boosting your cardiovascular fitness.

● **Play leapfrog.** You'll get a good leg and cardiovascular workout – and lots of fun. Everyone squats down low, imitating a frog on a lily pad. To leap over the person in front of you, place your hands on his or her back, then spring forward and up. Keep your legs and feet wide, in case you need to take two hops to clear your obstacle. Land with your knees soft and slightly bent to protect whoever's in front.

Play leapfrog with your children.

● **Challenge your children, grandchildren, partner or colleagues to a toe-walking contest every other day.** Rise onto the balls of your feet and walk across the room. Whoever lowers his or her heels to the floor first loses. You'll have plenty of laughs and strengthen your arches, ankles and calves.

● **Add a hill to your walking route.** As you trudge up, you'll feel the muscles in the backs of your legs working hard to push off with every step.

● **Practise 'hot seats' as you watch TV.** Television time doesn't have to be couch potato time. Pledge that you won't sit down on your favourite recliner until you've done 15 to 20 hot seats during the adverts. To do a hot seat, stand with your feet slightly wider than your hips. Sit back into a squat, just until your bottom touches the seat of the chair. As soon as you feel the seat of the chair under your bottom, spring up to a standing position, as if the seat were 'hot'.

☺ **Whenever you stand in a queue, balance on one foot.** As soon as you lift one foot off the ground, the muscles in the foot, ankle, calf, thigh and buttock of the opposite leg firm up as they work harder to keep you upright. If you're worried about what other people might think, balance on one foot – no one will notice.

☆ **Do a squat every time you pick something up off the floor.** Bending over to pick something up from the waist puts stress on the lower back, especially if you're lifting something heavy. But a squat forces you to use your legs, building up your leg strength. The best way to squat: with your feet hip-distance apart or wider, knees bent and your bottom stuck out as you squat down. Then bend forward and pick up your object. Bring your torso upright, then rise by pressing up through your heels. Even if you just squat to pick up a pencil, it will help you to build more leg strength.

● **Exercise your calf muscles while you brush your teeth.** Place your feet flat on the floor, then rise up onto the balls of your feet, hold for 2 seconds, and sink down. Repeat 20, 30, 50 or more times. You can do this not only while brushing your teeth, but any time you are waiting.

☆ **Push against immovable objects.** Isometric exercises are the best way to exercise without moving. Your goal: to put your foot or upper thigh against a surface that won't move or break, and to press against it hard (but not so hard as to strain your muscles or joints). Hold each position for 6 to 8 seconds, relax for a few seconds, then repeat five to ten times on each side.

NECK & SHOULDER strength

You might wonder why neck and shoulder strength matters. You're not training for a rugby team or pulling a plough. Yet strength in these areas is vital to your overall well-being. Neck pain, be it caused by bad sleep, bad posture or too much stress, is among the most common everyday complaints. Research shows that neck-strengthening exercises may be more important than stretching when it comes to preventing neck pain. The same goes for shoulder strength. Weak shoulders increase the stress on your elbows and wrists. Here are some simple ways to build neck and shoulder strength.

12 SIMPLE STRATEGIES THAT DECREASE PAIN AND STIFFNESS

● **Whenever you feel exasperated at work,** press your forehead into your palms. Many of us tense up our neck muscles when under stress, which can lead to pain and stiffness over time. You can reduce tension and strengthen your neck at the same time with this simple exercise.

● Sitting at your desk, lean forward and place your elbows on your desk. With your head centred over your shoulders, press your forehead into your palms, using your palms to resist the pressure of your head. Hold this position for 3 to 5 seconds, release and repeat three to five times. Now sit up straight and place your palms on the back of your head with your elbows out to the sides. Press your head back into your palms as you use your palms to resist the pressure of your head. Hold for 3 to 5 seconds, release, then repeat three to five times.

● **Boost yourself up twice a day.** Here's another great exercise for the office. Place your palms on the edge of your chair and press down into your hands, lifting your hips and bottom an inch or two into the air. Hold for 5 seconds, lower and repeat five times for a great shoulder muscle strengthener.

☆ **Hire a rowing boat** and take your partner for a romantic jaunt on a lake or pond. As you row out onto the water, you'll strengthen the weakest section of your shoulders, behind your shoulder blades. When these muscles are weak, your shoulders slump forward. If rowing's impractical, simulate the motion for a few minutes, moving slowly and carefully, with a piece of rubber tubing attached to a door handle. Or use a rowing machine at home or at the gym.

● **Practise shrugging your shoulders.** The action of lifting your shoulders up to your ears will strengthen your neck and shoulder muscles. For a fuller workout, do three sets of ten shrugs.

▶ **Make sure you're sleeping on the right pillow.** The best pillow for you depends on your own preferences, but generally stomach sleepers should go for soft, side sleepers for medium, and back sleepers for firm.

Do THREE things...

The repetitive movements involved in working at a computer all day – making micro-movement after micro-movement and staring at your screen for hours on end – can, over time, stiffen the muscles in your arms, shoulders and neck, causing pain. A number of treatments can be used to prevent and reverse 'computer neck', ranging from chiropractic manipulation to massage. Here are three tactics that have been proven by research to reduce neck pain, according to Claire Small of Pure Sports Medicine.

1 Exercise aerobically for at least 30 minutes three to four times a week. Regular aerobic exercise increases blood flow to your muscles, helping them to heal faster. A brisk walk works just fine.

2 Lose weight. Excess pounds not only encourage you to sit with poor posture, they also impede blood circulation, slowing the healing process. You can lose 1lb (0.5kg) a week by eliminating 250kcal a day from your diet and walking for 20 additional minutes a day.

3 Quit smoking. Research shows that smoking can cause all types of pain, including neck and back pain. The nicotine in tobacco is toxic to all body tissues and may damage the blood vessels in your neck and shoulders, preventing blood from getting to your spine.

Exercise your **ROTATOR CUFF**

● **Exercise your rotator cuff once a week.** Your rotator cuff is actually a group of muscles and tendons that holds your shoulder joint in place. Most people neglect to strengthen this area of the body because these deep muscles don't play much of a role in shaping sexy shoulder contours and, quite frankly, no one tells you about these muscles until after you've already injured them. Yet strengthening them will go a long way towards preventing shoulder problems later in life. You can do the following exercises at home.

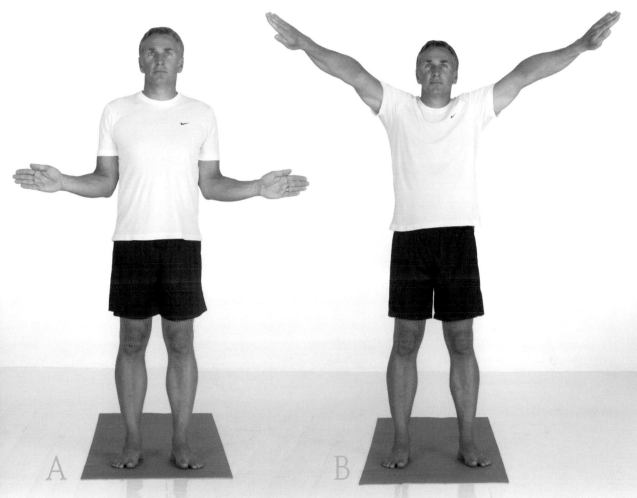

Stand with your elbows pressed into your waist, your upper arms snuggled next to your ribs, your elbows bent at 90 degrees, and your palms facing each other. Open your shoulders by pulling your shoulder blades together behind your back. Keeping your upper arms and elbows touching your sides, open your hands slowly out to your sides. You should feel tension between your shoulder blades. Hold for five, bring your palms together, and repeat ten times.

Stand with your feet under your hips and your arms at your sides. Raise your arms out to the sides and forward at an angle of 45 degrees to your torso as high as you can with your little fingers facing up. Keep your shoulders relaxed away from your ears as you raise your arms. Lower and repeat 10 to 20 times. As the exercise becomes easier, attach ankle weights to your wrists to increase the challenge.

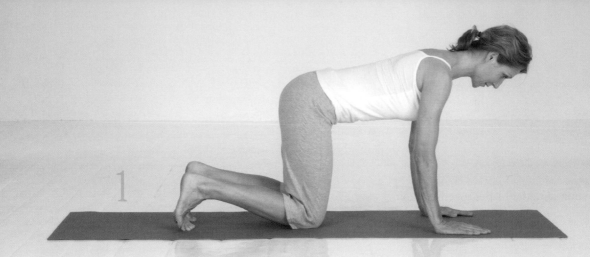

Morning STRETCH

● **Every morning before you get dressed, stretch into a yoga down dog.** This quintessential yoga posture stretches your calves, hamstrings, chest and spine, while it strengthens and stretches your shoulders. Kneel with your palms on the floor under your shoulders and knees under your hips. Spread your fingers as wide as you can, with your middle fingers pointing forward. Tuck your toes under, coming onto the balls of your feet. Roll your shoulder blades away from each other, bringing the creases of your elbows towards each other. Lift your tail bone (coccyx). Then exhale as you extend your legs and lift your hips towards the ceiling, forming an upside-down V shape with your body. Relax your head between your arms. Press into your palms to bring more body weight back into your legs. Continue to roll your shoulder blades away from each other and the inner creases of your elbows towards each other. Hold for five to ten breaths. Lower and repeat.

☺ **As you watch television at night, retract your shoulder blades.** Sit on the edge of your chair and lengthen your spine, as if you were trying to grow taller. Place your hands in your lap. Bring your shoulders as far back as you can, pinching your shoulder blades together. Hold for the length of an entire commercial. Relax, then repeat one more time during the course of the evening.

▐▶ **When you get home from work,** stuff a sock three-quarters full with white rice, 2 cinnamon sticks and 1 tablespoon of cloves. Seal the end tightly with a rubber band. Heat for 2 minutes in the microwave, then drape the sock around your neck for a surprisingly pleasing aromatherapeutic remedy for sore shoulders and neck. There's no need to empty the sock when you're finished – you can use it over and over, until the spices lose their fragrance.

● **Whenever you spend more than 45 minutes in the driver's seat or in front of the computer, practise the 'turtle' exercise.** Often during driving and when staring at a computer screen, we tend to jut our heads forward, as if sticking our nose out is going to get us to our destination faster or help us to finish that project quicker. Because the head weighs about 4.5kg, this puts quite a bit of stress on the back of the neck. Before you know it, you've got a headache. You can both strengthen the muscles in the back of your neck and train yourself to sit with proper posture with the following exercise. As you drive or type, pretend you're a turtle retracting your head into your shell. Keeping your chin level, bring your head back, flattening the curve in the back of your neck. Hold for a count of five, release, and repeat ten times.

● **Every hour, drop your chin to your chest,** then roll your neck to the left, back, to the right and down again in a circular motion. Repeat five times, then switch direction, starting with a roll to the right.

● **Start each working day with a chair exercise.** Sit on the edge of a chair with your knees bent and feet on the floor. Extend one arm overhead and the other towards the floor, with your palms facing in. Keeping your shoulders low on your back and away from your ears, reach back through both arms, feeling a stretch through your top armpit and front of your lower shoulder. You'll also feel muscles in the backs of your shoulders and upper back firming up as they work to keep your arms in place. Hold for 2 seconds, then switch positions, so the top arm is now facing towards the floor and the bottom arm is facing the ceiling, and repeat. Continue to hold for 2 seconds, then switch positions 20 times. Then do the same movement 20 times, but turn your hands so that your palms face behind your torso. Finally, repeat the exercise again, but turn your hands so that your palms face forward. Each new palm position strengthens and stretches a slightly different area of your shoulders.

SELF-MASSAGE

Have you ever had a professional massage? If you have, you know what a terrific experience it is. A massage helps to reduce muscle tension in many ways, including increasing blood flow to your muscles. Some research shows that having a regular massage may also boost your immunity by stimulating the production of white blood cells. Not only that, a massage may also make you more productive at work. Researchers have found that a brief self-massage at work reduced stress and boosted job performance. Fortunately, you have your very own massage therapist with you at all times – your hands! The tips that follow give you advice on how to reduce tension from head to foot.

16 WAYS TO REDUCE TENSION IN SECONDS

☆ **Every morning and evening, hammer out the kinks.** Using your fists, gently thump the outside of your body, starting with your legs and arms, working from top to bottom. Then move inwards to your torso and thump from bottom to top. Pummelling your muscles and bones will help to strengthen your body, stimulate blood circulation and relax nerve endings. If you do it in the morning, this self-massage technique will waken and prepare your body – and mind – for the day ahead. When done before bed, it calms down the mind and beats out the stress and tension of the day. One warning: don't do this if you're taking any kind of blood thinner, such as warfarin; you could end up with bruising.

● **Rub your stomach after every meal.** Most of us do this instinctively, especially after overeating. Place one or both palms on your abdomen and rub it in clockwise circles. This is the same direction that food naturally moves through your intestine, so your circular massage will help to stimulate digestion.

☺ **Rub yourself down before and after exercise.** Massaging your body before your stretching, cardio or strength training increases blood flow to the muscles. Massaging your muscles after exercise may help to encourage waste removal and speed muscle recovery. Before exercise, use a pummelling motion with your fists to bring blood flow to your leg and arm muscles. After exercise, rub along your muscles with your palm or fist, moving in the direction of your heart.

● **Give your hands a massage every day** – whenever you put on lotion. Start with the bottom of your palms by clasping your fingers and rubbing the heels of your palms together in a circular motion.

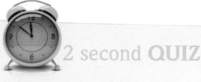

2 second **QUIZ**

Hard or soft massage?
ANSWER: **HARD.**

The point of massage isn't to stimulate the skin; it's to relieve the muscles lying deep below the skin. While you're not advised to massage to the point of pain, you need to use enough effort to work the muscles thoroughly. And that takes more force than many home massagers assert. If your hands and arms aren't getting strained or tired giving a massage, you're probably not pressing hard enough.

Then, with your hands still clasped, take one thumb and massage the area just below your other thumb in circular motions, moving outwards to the centre of the palm. Repeat with the other hand. Then release your fingers and use your thumbs and index fingers to knead your palms, wrists and the webbing between your fingers. With one hand, gently pull each finger of the other hand. Finish by using your thumb and index finger to pinch the webbing between your other thumb and index finger.

● **Roll on a tennis ball to release tension.** If your foot feels tense, stand with one hand on a wall for support and place the arch of the foot on top of the ball. Gradually add more body weight over the foot, allowing the ball to press into your arch. Begin to move your foot slowly, allowing the ball to massage your heel, forefoot and toes. If the tennis ball seems too big for your foot, try a golf ball instead.

You can also lie on the ball to get at that hard-to-reach spot between the shoulder blades or to soothe tension in your lower back. For tight hips, sit on the ball, wiggling your bottom around and holding it in any spot that feels good.

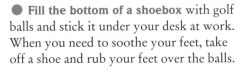

The secret of happy feet is a hidden box of golf balls.

● **Fill the bottom of a shoebox** with golf balls and stick it under your desk at work. When you need to soothe your feet, take off a shoe and rub your feet over the balls.

● **Whenever you take off a pair of high heels,** sit on the floor and give your calves some attention. Elevating your heels all day long can eventually shorten your calf muscles. To release them, sit with your knees bent and feet on the floor. Grasp one ankle, placing your thumb just above your Achilles tendon. Press your thumb into the bottom of your calf muscle, hold for 5 seconds, then release. Move an inch up your calf and repeat the pressure. Continue pressing and releasing until you get to your knee, then switch legs.

● **Use your hands to *heel* your neck.** Once an hour, take a break and clasp your fingers behind your neck, pressing the heels of your palms into your neck on either side of your spine. Massage the heels of your hands up and down in slow, deliberate motions. Then place the fingers of your right hand on your trapezius muscle along the left side of your neck just below the base of your skull. Press into that muscle, tilt your head to the left and rub downwards until you reach your shoulder. Repeat three times, then swap

sides. Finish by stretching your head back so that the top of your office chair presses into your neck just below your skull. This also stretches out the front of your neck, which tends to get tight during desk work. Hold for 20 seconds.

● **Make congested sinuses more comfortable with some finger pressure.** If you have clogged sinuses due to a cold or allergies, rub them with your index fingers. Start just above your brow line. Place your finger pads just above your nose, press down and rub outwards, tracing your brow line as you go. Repeat two or three times. Then place the pads of your fingers below your eyes and to the sides of the bridge of your nose, rubbing outwards and moving downwards with each stroke. Now use your thumbs to massage your cheekbones, making small circles starting at the centre of your face and moving out towards your ears. Finally, place your thumbs on your temples and massage them in small circles.

● **When your eyes feel tired** from staring at your computer screen all day long, give them some heat. Rub your hands together vigorously until you feel the skin on your palms begin to warm up. Then cup one hand over each eye, feeling the heat from your hands relax your eyes.

☺ **If your feet are sore after a long day** of standing, take off your shoes and socks, wash your feet and give them a rub-down. Sitting on a comfortable couch or chair, thread the fingers of one hand through the toes of one foot, spreading out your toes and placing the palm of your hand against the bottom of your foot. Use your palm to rotate the joints of your forefoot forward and back gently for 1 minute. Then remove your fingers from your toes, hold your ankle with one hand, and gently rotate the entire foot with the other hand, starting with small circles and progressing to larger circles as your ankle warms up. Switch directions, then repeat with the other foot.

● **Give yourself a bear-hug to relax away shoulder tension.** Cross your arms over your chest and grab a shoulder with either hand. Squeeze each shoulder and release three times. Then move your hands down your arms, squeezing and releasing until you get to your wrists.

⭐ **Rub lavender oil onto your feet before you go to bed.** Lavender-scented oils are available at most health-food shops. The smell of lavender and the gentle massaging motions you make as you work the oil into your feet will help you to unwind. An added bonus: the nightly oil treatment softens and hydrates any rough, dry spots on your feet. Once you've finished your massage, put on a pair of socks to prevent the oil from rubbing off onto your sheets.

● **After tennis, cycling, rock climbing,** and other arm-tiring sports, give your arms a pinch. Place your right arm across your chest with your elbow bent. Reach across your chest with your left arm and pinch your right arm's triceps, near the shoulder, with the thumb and index

finger of your left hand. Hold for a few seconds, release, then pinch again an inch lower on the arm. Continue pinching and releasing until you've made your way to your elbow. Then pinch your right arm's biceps near your armpit and work your way in the same way down to the elbow. Then switch arms. This will release the tension in your muscles and help to improve blood circulation.

● **When you have a headache,** stand up, bend forward from the hips and place your forehead on a padded chair. The chair will gently place pressure on your head as you relax in the forward bend. Hold for about 30 seconds. When you rise, sit down and spread your fingers through your hair, making a fist. Gently pull the hair away from your head. Hold for 2 or 3 seconds, then release. This stretches the fascia, the fibrous tissue, along your scalp, releasing tension. Continue to grab different clumps of hair all over your head, working from the top front of your head, progressing to the sides, and then to the back. Once you have grabbed and released your entire scalp, return to work refreshed.

● **Keep a tennis ball on your desk and squeeze it regularly.** The squeezing motion helps to rejuvenate tired fingers and hands, and strengthens your hands for other self-massage techniques.

Reminder

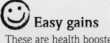**Fast results**
These are tips that deliver benefits particularly quickly – in some cases, immediately.

☺ **Easy gains**
These are health boosters that offer the best value for the least amount of effort.

⭐ **Super-effective**
This is advice that scientific research or widespread usage by experts has shown to be especially effective.

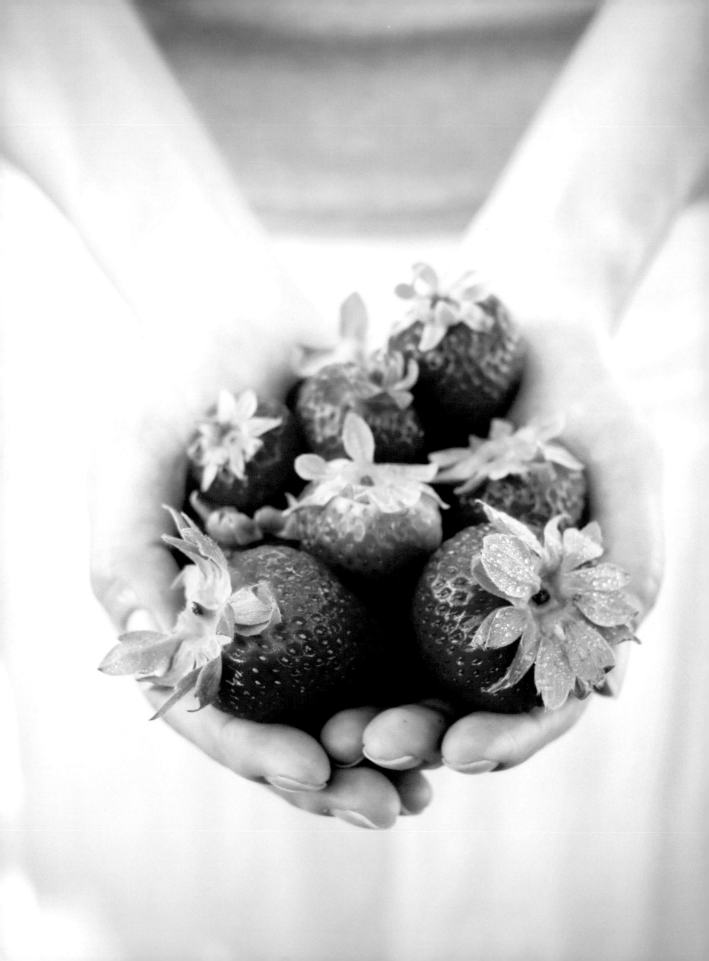

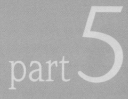

part 5

HEALTH GOALS

As we travel through life, each of us encounters unique health challenges and concerns. To help you make your journey as disease – and worry – free as possible, we've put together proven health tips for 18 common health goals, from losing weight to preventing cancer.

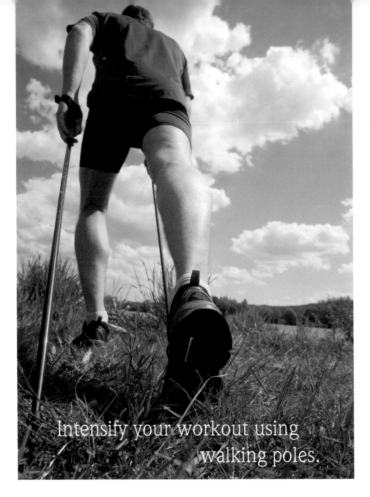

Intensify your workout using walking poles.

order a fancy calorie-packed frappuccino. And skip the espresso if it makes you toss and turn at night.

● **Don't worry if you've been yo-yo dieting.** There's a myth that if you've spent your life losing and gaining the same 10 to 20lb (4.5 to 9kg), your metabolism gets out of kilter and ends up slowing right down. Don't believe it. When researchers reviewed 43 studies on the topic, they found no difference in the metabolic rates of yo-yo dieters compared to those of everyone else.

● **Walk with intent – and intensity.** Burn more calories in the same amount of time with these strategies:
● Swing your arms when you walk. You'll burn 5 to 10 per cent more calories.
● Wear a weighted vest – another great way to burn calories. But leave the hand and ankle weights at home. They throw you off balance and could result in injury.
● Walk on grass, sand or a gravel path instead of the road. It takes more muscle power to glide smoothly over these uneven surfaces (especially sand) than over tarmac.
● Use walking poles. A US study found that you get a much more intense workout than you would without the poles.
● Walk along the shoreline of a beach, lake or pond with your ankles in the water. The resistance burns more calories and gives your muscles an added workout.

● **Increase the protein in your diet.** There is some evidence that if you increase your protein intake to the upper end of the recommended range (roughly 20 per cent of overall calories), the amount of energy you expend at rest will remain the same even while you're losing weight. Normally, as you lose weight, your body adjusts and you burn fewer calories at rest.

● Exercise outside. Maybe it's the fresh air, maybe it's the sunshine, but something about exercising out in the open makes you walk or run faster than doing the same exercise in the gym.

☺ **Eat five small meals throughout the day instead of three large meals.** You might think you should eat less often if you want to lose weight, but that's just not the case. By eating every few hours, you keep your metabolism fired up and ensure it doesn't slow down between meals in order to hang on to calories. A 'meal' can be as small as a cup of soup.

● **Sip a couple of cups of coffee throughout the day.** Studies find that the caffeine in coffee increases the rate at which your body burns calories. This does not mean, however, that you should

LOSING weight

If you're overweight, one of the best things you can do for your overall health is lose a few pounds. Or maybe more than a few pounds. Carrying too much weight significantly increases your risk of heart disease, diabetes, stroke, high blood pressure, cancer ... the list seems almost endless. Plus, if you do fall ill or need surgery, being overweight can make any treatments riskier.

You know the drill by now when it comes to losing weight – take in fewer calories than you burn off. But you probably also know that most diets and quick weight-loss plans are not really sustainable. You're better off finding several simple things you can do on a daily basis – and following the cardinal rules of eating more fruit and vegetables and less fat while making sure you get more physical activity.

Together with our tips, these actions should send the numbers on your scales in the right direction: down.

47 OF THE BEST TIPS FOR EASY SLIMMING

Greater ENERGY

Do you find yourself collapsing on the couch by midafternoon? Are you feeling more sluggish than a hungover sloth? Do you envy the boundless energy of your children or grandchildren – or even your on-the-go next-door neighbour? Don't blame your age; blame your lifestyle. A low-energy lifestyle leaves you with little energy. A high-energy lifestyle gives you lots of energy. For most people, it's that simple.

Indeed, with just a few easy changes to your daily routine, it's guaranteed that the seemingly permanent imprint of your bottom on the sofa will rise up and vanish, along with your inertia.

Your friends and family may start asking what you're taking. Tell them nothing, except some good health-boosting advice.

23 WAYS TO FIND YOUR GET UP AND GO AFTER IT HAS GOT UP AND GONE

✪ **Nurse a coffee throughout the day.** If you need a quadruple shot of espresso just to bring your eyelids to half mast in the morning, you may be driving yourself deeper and deeper into a low-energy rut. Compelling research from various institutions, including Harvard Medical School, finds that frequent low doses of caffeine – the amount in a quarter-cup of coffee – are more effective than a few larger doses of caffeine in keeping people alert.

✪ **Lighten your glycaemic load.** Foods with a low glycaemic load (see page 100) – such as beans, bran cereal, brown rice, wholemeal bread and nuts – have less impact on your blood sugar than foods with a high glycaemic load – including white rice, spaghetti, potatoes, cornflakes and sugary juices and drinks. Eating more low glycaemic-load foods will help you to keep your blood sugar steady and avoid the lightheadedness and 'shakes' associated with blood sugar drops, which usually follow rises.

✪ **If you have dried rosemary in your kitchen, crush a small handful and take a whiff or three.** The herb's intense woody fragrance is known to herbalists as an invigorating stimulant.

☆ **Once a day, try to go for a 10 minute 'thank you' walk.** As you walk, focus your thoughts on the things for which you feel most thankful. After the walk, make a mental note of how you feel. This simple technique gives you both a sense of wellbeing and the positive benefits of walking and exercise, flooding your brain with happy neurotransmitters and endorphins. It's simple, yet it's a powerful exercise that energises the mind and body, and builds mental and physical muscle.

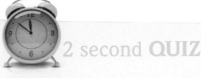

2 second QUIZ

Cup of coffee or 20 minute nap?
ANSWER: **A NAP.**

This is according to a French review of research on techniques that helped night-shift workers to remain alert. Set an alarm to wake you in 20 minutes. A longer nap could interfere with your sleep later that night.

✪ **When you find yourself thinking a negative thought, picture a stop sign.** Then either push the thought out of your mind or replace it with a positive one. Negative feelings take a lot of mental energy. Whenever possible, avoid unnecessary self-criticism. Stop blaming yourself for past events that you cannot change. You deserve the same level of respect and kindness as others.

▐▐▶ **Drink two glasses of icy water.** Fatigue is often one of the first symptoms of dehydration, and if all you've sipped throughout the day is coffee and soft drinks, it's quite likely that you're dehydrated. Plus, the refreshing coldness will serve as a virtual slap in the face.

✪ **Soak a flannel in icy water and place it over your face.** The icy coolness of the cloth will quickly rejuvenate your facial muscles and eyes. It will probably lift your spirits as well.

✪ **Get enough iron.** Constantly dragging yourself around? You could have iron-deficiency anaemia, a common cause of fatigue. Iron is essential for producing haemoglobin, which carries oxygen to your body's cells, where it's used to produce energy. Good food sources of iron are red meat, iron-fortified breakfast

Eat something crunchy.

⚽ **Turn off the news for one week.** Depressing television news of murders, fires and terrorism can quickly drain your mental reserves. If you're a news junkie, try this experiment for one week: stop reading your newspaper and watch only one television news programme a day (or none if you can stand it). Notice how you feel at the end of the week. If you feel more energetic and peaceful, stick to your new habit.

⚽ **List all the people you're angry with and write a friendly letter to each one.** Brooding over past events only drains your energy. Try to accept others for who they are and don't expend a lot of effort on changing them. You don't have to send the letter. Simply writing it is enough.

⚽ **Soak up a little sun in winter.** Do you have all the energy of a hibernating bear in winter months? Make a point of getting outside for 30 minutes to an hour during the day. The natural light can improve your energy levels and help to fight seasonal affective disorder (SAD).

☺ **In the hour before bedtime, turn off the TV,** put away your work and relax with a good book, some embroidery or a crossword puzzle. Take a warm bath and listen to soothing music. This ritual will help you to fall asleep more quickly and experience a more restful slumber, resulting in a more energetic you the following day.

⚽ **Create an area for sorting out the post.** Clutter is not only distracting, it's frustrating and energy-wasting. (How many times have you scoured the house for lost keys or bills that were right in front of you?) To keep track of your bills and other post, buy an open box file or some hanging files from an office supply

cereal, green leafy vegetables and all beans and pulses. You may also need a supplement; check with your doctor.

⚽ **When someone asks you to do something, say,** 'Let me check my diary and I'll get back to you.' This gives you time to think about the request and decide if it's something you really want to do, or simply an energy-sucking waste of your time. Don't overextend yourself, especially doing tasks you don't really enjoy. If you don't want to bake for another school fete, say so.

⚽ **Have your thyroid checked.** If it's not producing enough thyroid hormone, it could be making you feel tired and rundown. A simple blood test will show if that's the case. Other symptoms of low thyroid are dry skin, weight gain, constipation and feeling cold.

shop. Place it in your kitchen and use it to sort your post into categories such as bills, receipts and letters.

⚽ **Breathe in new energy.** Sit in a chair with a straight back. Place your hands over your stomach and breathe into your tummy so that your hands rise and fall with your breath. Imagine you're inhaling a white light that fills your body with vital energy. Do this for five full breaths. Then, as you inhale, tighten the muscles that connect your shoulders and neck, pulling your shoulders up towards your ears. When you've inhaled all you can and your shoulders are snug around your ears, hold your breath for just a second. Then exhale as you release the tension and your breath in one big whoosh – as if you were releasing the weight of the world from your shoulders. Repeat until you feel clear, refreshed and revitalised.

⚽ **Make a list of everything you're looking forward to in the next month.** Do this every month when you pay your rent or mortgage. Simply building more anticipation into your life helps to stoke up your energy.

▶ **Eat something crunchy.** Pretzels, carrots and other crunchy foods make your jaw work hard, which can wake up your facial muscles, helping you to feel more alert.

⚽ **Chew a piece of peppermint or spearmint chewing gum.** You'll get a burst of energy from the invigorating flavour and scent, not to mention the physical act of chewing.

⚽ **Eat every 4 hours.** It's much better to refuel your body continually before it hits empty than to wait until you're in the danger zone then overdo it. So every

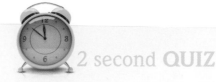

2 second QUIZ

Yoga or aerobic exercise?
ANSWER: **EITHER.**

In a study of patients with multiple sclerosis, yoga and stationary cycling improved energy levels to the same degree. Just pick one and do it.

4 hours (except, of course, when you're sleeping), have a mini-meal or snack. A mini-meal might be a handful of roasted peanuts, a hard-boiled egg or a slice of lean cold meat and a sliced apple. Fat-free yoghurt sprinkled with linseeds makes a good, nutritious snack.

⚽ **Stay still.** You wouldn't think stillness would lead to energy, but often that's just what you need to create your second wind. Simply sit for 10 minutes in a comfortable chair and stare out of the window. Let your mind drift wherever it wants to go. Allow yourself just to 'be', something we're often too frenzied to do.

⚽ **Or stretch.** Stand up, get on your toes and lift your fingertips as close as you can to the ceiling. Keep the stretch expanding for several seconds, feeling it in your calves, your abdomen, your shoulders, your arms, your fingers. After a few seconds, relax, take a few deep breaths and do it again. By doing this, you activate almost every muscle you have, sending oxygen-rich blood throughout your body.

⚽ **Make a list of every relationship in your life** and rank how those relationships make you feel, from 1 (terrible) to 5 (fabulous). Bad relationships are known energy sappers. Take note of the relationships that don't add any positive energy, and develop plans to remove yourself adroitly from them.

MONITOR
your health

Many of us go for regular check-ups and blood tests. But that's not to say that in between visits you should close your eyes and cross your fingers that all's still well. The fact is that while your doctor may see you once or twice a year, you live in your body every single day, and that makes you the best judge of your own health – if you know what clues to look for. Here are 15 ways to play doctor detective.

15 WAYS TO DO IT WITHOUT A DOCTOR

☆ **Have a PERF-ect day.** Essentially, there are four things you should monitor every day to make sure you are living healthily: the amount of fruit and vegetables you ate that day (fresh Produce); whether you walked and were active (Exercise); whether you got at least 15 minutes of laughter and fun time for yourself (Relaxation); and whether you got enough beans, grains and other high-fibre foods (Fibre). If you can say you did well on all four, your day has been extremely healthy.

☆ **Monitor your sleepiness.** There are three good ways to tell if you're getting enough sleep. First, do you require an alarm clock to wake up most mornings? Second, do you become drowsy in the afternoon to the point that it affects what you're doing? Third, do you doze off shortly after eating dinner? If the answer to any of these is yes, you need more sleep. And if you're getting enough sleep (about 8 hours) and still have these troubles, talk to your doctor about your low energy.

● **Check your hairbrush.** If your hair's falling out, ask your doctor to check your levels of blood ferritin, an indication of how much iron your body is storing. Some studies suggest low levels may be related to unexplained hair loss. Thyroid disease is another fairly common cause.

● **Measure your height every year after you turn 50.** This is especially important for women as a way of assessing posture and skeletal health. A change in stature can be as informative as a change on a bone density test in terms of assessing your overall bone health. If you're concerned, ask your GP about having a bone density test: it picks up bone loss even before your height changes.

Healthy INVESTMENT

● **Keep a mental colour chart of how dark your urine is.** It may sound weird, but it's a useful health indicator. Your urine should be a clear, straw colour; if it's dark or smells strong, you may not be getting enough fluids. If it stays dark-coloured even after you increase your liquid intake, make an appointment to see your doctor. If it's bright yellow, it may be the B vitamins in your multivitamin.

● **Check your heartbeat after you exercise.** A study published in the *Journal of the American Medical Association* found that women with poor heart rate recovery (HRR) after exercise had twice the risk of having a heart attack within ten years as those who had normal HRR. To test your HRR after regular strenuous activity, count your heartbeats for 15 seconds, then multiply by four to get your heart rate. Sit down and wait 2 minutes before checking again. Subtract the second number from the first. If it's under 55, your HRR is higher than normal and you should talk it through with your doctor.

Your hairbrush may provide valuable health clues.

PREVENTING
colds and flu

When you're deep under the covers with a box of tissues by your bedside do you turn green with envy thinking of those people who never seem to get ill? Want to be one of them? While colds won't kill you, they can weaken your immune system, allowing other, more serious, germs to take hold. Given that most of us have two or three colds a year, that's a lot of opportunities for serious illness. Although it's impossible to promise that you'll never catch another cold or suffer from another bout of flu, you can increase your odds of staying well with these strategies. And if you do become ill, there are some tips on how to get better faster.

22 WAYS TO STAY HEALTHY ALL YEAR ROUND

Wash your hands and wash them often. A US study of 40,000 naval recruits who were ordered to wash their hands five times a day found that the recruits cut their incidence of respiratory illnesses by 45 per cent.

● **Every time you wash your hands, do it twice.** Researchers who looked for germs on volunteers' hands found that one handwashing had little effect, even when using antibacterial soap. So wash twice if you're serious about fending off colds.

● **Use this hand-drying strategy in public toilets.** Studies find a shockingly large percentage of people fail to wash their hands after using a public toilet. And every single one of them touches the door handle on the way out. So after washing your hands, use a paper towel to turn off the tap. Use another paper towel to dry your hands, then open the door with that paper towel as a barrier between you and the handle. It sounds a bit crazy, but it could help to protect you from infectious diseases such as colds and flu.

☺ **Carry hand sanitiser with you.** Colds are typically passed not from coughing or kissing (although those are two modes of transmission) but from hand-to-hand or hand-to-object contact, since most cold viruses can live for hours on objects. You then put your hand in or near your mouth or nose and, voilà, you're infected. Carry hand sanitiser gel or sanitising wipes with you and you can clean your hands at any time, even if the closest water supply is miles away. It works.

● **Use your knuckle to rub your eyes.** It's less likely to be contaminated with viruses than your fingertip. This is particularly important given that the eye provides a perfect entry point for germs, and most of us rub our eyes or nose or scratch our faces 20 to 50 times a day.

● **Put your toothbrush in the microwave** on high for 10 seconds to kill germs that can cause colds and other illnesses. Once you're finished brushing your teeth, your toothbrush is a breeding ground for germs. Sterilise it in the microwave before you use it or simply replace it every month when you change the page on your calendar and after you've had a cold.

☆ **Get a flu vaccination every autumn.** Flu vaccination is generally offered free of charge on the NHS to everyone over 65, and to anyone with a long-term medical problem that makes them more vulnerable (for example, heart or lung disease, being on immunosuppressant drugs, having diabetes or no spleen). Employers should also offer the vaccine to health-care staff.

● **Stop blaming yourself when things go wrong at work.** Believe it or not, blaming yourself makes you more likely to catch a cold. At least, that's what researchers found when they studied more than 200 workers over three months. Even those who had control over their work were more likely to begin sneezing if they lacked confidence or tended to blame themselves when things went wrong. Researchers believe that such attitudes make people more stressed on the job, and stress, as everyone knows, can challenge your immune system.

> Microwave your toothbrush to eradicate nasty germs.

☺ **Leave the windows in your house open a crack in winter.** Not all of them, but one or two in the rooms in which you spend the most time. This is particularly important if you live in a newer home, if fresh circulating air has been sacrificed to energy efficiency. A bit of fresh air will do wonders for chasing out germs.

● **Lower the heat in your house by a few degrees.** The dry air of an overheated home provides the perfect environment for cold viruses to thrive. And when your mucous membranes (of the nose, mouth and tonsils) dry out, they can't trap those germs very well. Lowering the temperature and using a room humidifier helps to maintain a healthier level of humidity in winter.

● **Speaking of which, buy a hygrometer.** These little tools measure humidity. You want the reading in your home to be around 50 per cent. A consistent measure higher than 60 per cent means mould and mildew may start to grow on your walls, fabrics and kitchen; lower than 40 per cent and the dry air makes you more susceptible to germs.

● **Sit in a sauna once a week.** Why? Because an Austrian study published in 1990 found that volunteers who frequently used a sauna had half as many colds during the six month study period as those who didn't use a sauna at all. It's possible that the hot air you inhale kills cold viruses. Most gyms have saunas these days.

☆ **Take a garlic supplement every day.** When 146 volunteers received either one garlic supplement a day or a placebo for 12 weeks between November and February, those taking the garlic were not only less likely to get a cold, but if they did catch one, their symptoms were less intense and they recovered faster.

● **Eat a pot of yoghurt every day.** A study by an American university found that people who ate one pot of yoghurt – whether live culture or pasteurised – had 25 per cent fewer colds than non-yoghurt eaters. Start your yoghurt eating in the summer to build up your immunity before the cold and flu season starts.

● **Once a day, sit in a quiet, dim room,** close your eyes and focus on one word. You're meditating, which is a proven way of reducing stress. And stress, studies find, increases your susceptibility to colds. In fact, stressed people have up to twice the number of colds as non-stressed people.

● **Scrub under your fingernails** every night. They're a great hiding place for all sorts of germs.

Eating a pot of yoghurt every day may chase away any sniffles.

● **Change or wash your hand towels** every three or four days during the cold and flu season. When you wash them, use hot water in order to kill the germs.

☆ **At the very first hint of a cold, launch a preventive blitz. Here's how:**
● Suck on a zinc lozenge until it melts away. Then suck another every two waking hours. Or use a zinc-based nasal spray. Some studies suggest that zinc may help, but the jury is still out.
● Cook up a pot of chicken soup.
● Roast garlic in the oven (drizzle whole cloves with olive oil, wrap in foil, roast for an hour at 200°C/gas mark 6), then spread the soft garlic on toast and eat.

Studies find that all either reduce the length of time you suffer from a cold or help to prevent a full-blown cold from occurring.

● **Sneeze and cough into your arm or into a tissue.** Whoever taught us to cover our mouths when we cough or sneeze got it wrong. That just puts the germs right on our hands, where you can spread them to objects – and other people. Instead, hold the crook of your elbow over your mouth and nose when you sneeze or cough if a tissue isn't handy. It's pretty rare for you to shake someone's elbow or scratch your eye with an elbow, after all.

● **Don't pressurise your doctor for antibiotics.** Colds and flu (along with most common infections) are caused by viruses, so antibiotics – designed to kill bacteria – won't do a thing. They can cause harm, however, by killing off the friendly bacteria that are part of our immune defences. If you've used antibiotics a lot lately, consider a course of probiotics – the replacement troops for friendly bacteria.

● **Wipe your nose – don't blow.** Your cold won't hang around as long, according to a US study. It turns out that the force of blowing not only sends the phlegm out of your nose into a tissue, but propels some back into your sinuses. If you need to blow, blow gently, and blow one nostril at a time.

● **Put a box of tissues wherever people sit.** In October, bulk buy boxes of tissues and place them strategically around the house, your workplace, your car. Don't let aesthetics thwart you. You need to have tissues widely available so that anyone who has to cough or sneeze or blow his or her nose will do so in the way that's least likely to spread germs.

Place a handy box of tissues wherever people sit and they're more likely to use them.

Reduce your risk of
HEART DISEASE
and STROKE

Death rates from cardiovascular disease (CVD) have been falling in the UK since the late 1970s. For people aged under 75, CVD rates have fallen by 40 per cent since 1998. And death rates from stroke also fell in the latter part of the 20th century. Good news? Well, a major factor in all this has been the advances of modern medicine. But is your idea of a healthy future being pulled back from the brink by bypass surgery? Or needing a vast array of medicines? Far preferable is avoiding CVD altogether. Add these small changes to your life for a powerful dose of heart disease prevention.

25 SIMPLE SOLUTIONS

♥ **Ride your bike for 20 minutes a day.** When German researchers asked 100 men with mild chest pain, or angina, either to exercise for 20 minutes a day on a stationary bike or to undergo an artery-clearing procedure called angioplasty, they found that a year after the angioplasty, 21 men suffered a heart attack, stroke or other problem compared to only six of the bikers. Just remember: if you already have angina, you should begin an exercise programme only under medical supervision.

☆ **Eat a piece of dark chocolate several times a week.** Believe it or not, several small studies suggest that dark chocolate could be good for your heart. The beneficial effects are probably due to chemicals in chocolate called flavonoids, which help the arteries to stay flexible. Other properties of the sweet stuff seem to make arteries less likely to clot and prevent the 'bad' cholesterol, LDL, from oxidising, making it less likely to form plaque. Dark chocolate is also rich in magnesium. But steer clear of milk chocolate, which is high in butterfat and thus tends to raise cholesterol.

♥ **Have a beer once a day.** A study published in the *Journal of Agricultural and Food Chemistry* found that men who drank one beer a day for a month lowered their cholesterol levels, increased their blood levels of heart-healthy antioxidants and reduced their levels of fibrinogen, a protein that contributes to blood clots. Of course, red wine might be even better (see page 225). Choose either beer or wine – don't have both.

♥ **Record yourself at night.** If you hear yourself snoring (or if your sleeping partner has been kicking you a lot), make an appointment with your doctor. You may have sleep apnoea, a condition in which the breathing stops hundreds of times throughout the night. It can lead to high blood pressure and other medical problems, and even increase your risk of a heart attack or stroke.

♥ **Go to bed an hour earlier tonight.** A Harvard study of 70,000 women found that those who got less than 7 hours of sleep had a slightly higher risk of heart disease. Researchers suspect that lack of sleep increases stress hormones, raises blood pressure and affects blood sugar levels. Keep your overall sleeping time to no more than 9 hours, however. The same study found that women sleeping 9 or more hours had a slightly increased risk of heart disease.

☆ **Eat fish at least once a week.** Have it grilled, sautéed, baked or roasted. A study published in the *Journal of the American Medical Association* in April 2002 found that women who ate fish at least once a week were a third less likely to have a heart attack or die of heart disease than those who ate fish only once a month. Other studies show similar benefits for men. Another major study found that regular fish consumption reduced the risk of atrial fibrillation – rapid, irregular heartbeat – a major cause of sudden death.

♥ **Have a high-fibre breakfast cereal at least four times a week.** In a study published in the *American Journal of Clinical Nutrition* in September 1999, Harvard University scientists found that women who ate 23g of fibre a day – mostly from cereal – were 23 per cent less likely to have heart attacks than those who consumed only 11g of fibre. In men, a high-fibre diet slashed the chances of a heart attack by 36 per cent.

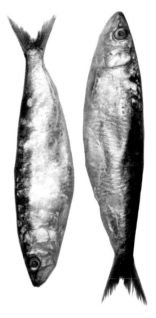

Keep your heart happy by eating fish at least once a week.

♥ **Cook with ginger or turmeric twice a week.** They have anti-inflammatory properties, and inflammation is a major contributor to heart disease.

♥ **Go to the loo whenever you feel the urge.** Research at Taiwan University found that a full bladder causes your heart to beat faster and puts added stress on the coronary arteries, triggering them to contract, which could lead to a heart attack in people who are vulnerable.

♥ **Ask for next Monday and Friday off.** American researchers analysed data on more than 12,000 middle-aged men from the famous Framingham Heart Study and found that those who took regular holidays sliced their risk of death from heart disease by a third.

♥ **Drive with the windows closed and the air-conditioning on.** This reduces your exposure to airborne pollutants, which a Harvard study found reduces something called 'heart rate variability' (HRV), or the ability of your heart to respond to various activities and stresses. Reduced HRV has been associated with increased deaths among heart attack survivors.

Man's best friend may also be your heart's best friend.

♥ **Call a friend and arrange dinner.** A study published in the journal *Heart* in April 2004 found that having a very close relationship with another person, whether it's a friend, lover or relative, can halve the risk of a heart attack in someone who has already had one.

♥ **Pay attention to the basics.** Two major studies published in 2003 found that nearly everyone who dies of heart disease, including heart attacks, had at least one or more of the conventional risk factors, such as smoking, diabetes, high blood pressure or high cholesterol levels.

☆ **Along with exercising every day, take a supplement** containing the amino acid L-arginine and the antioxidant vitamins C and E. A study published in the *Proceedings of the National Academy of Sciences* found that while moderate exercise alone reduced the development of atherosclerosis, or hardening of the arteries, adding L-arginine and the vitamins to the mix boosted the effects astronomically. The two – exercise and the supplements – have a synergistic effect in enhancing production of nitric oxide, which protects against a variety of heart-related problems.

♥ **If you find you're having trouble getting out of bed in the morning,** have lost interest in your normal activities, or just feel really off-colour, call your doctor. You may be depressed, and untreated depression significantly increases your risk of a heart attack.

♥ **Adopt a dog.** The power of furry friends to improve heart health is proven. Not only will a dog force you to be more active (think about all the walkies), but the companionship and unconditional affection a dog provides has been shown to reduce the risk of heart attack and other cardiovascular problems.

Lower your
CHOLESTEROL

About 70 per cent of UK adults have high cholesterol levels – now recognised as a significant health risk. If you're one of these people, it means that your body produces too much harmful low-density lipoprotein (LDL) but produces too little 'good' high-density lipoprotein (HDL). 'Bad' LDL carries cholesterol into your arteries, contributing to artery-clogging plaque and increasing the risk of heart disease and stroke, while 'good' HDL carries cholesterol away to the liver and out of the body.

You may already be taking cholesterol-lowering medication but you should still pay special attention to the tips in this chapter because diet can help to balance LDL and HDL and regulate your cholesterol levels. Research also suggests that by eating the right foods and taking good care of yourself, you could slash your risk of dying from heart disease by an incredible 80 per cent.

15 WAYS TO GET THE NUMBERS DOWN

What causes
HIGH CHOLESTEROL?

One of the main causes of high cholesterol levels in the blood in the UK is eating too much saturated fat. Here are some other cholesterol facts to be aware of:

● Although cholesterol is found in some foods such as eggs, liver, kidneys and some seafood, such as prawns, this type of cholesterol generally does not affect the cholesterol levels in your blood. It is more important to tackle the amount of saturated fat you consume, and to replace saturated and trans fats with healthier monounsaturated and polyunsaturated fats.

● Some people who eat a healthy diet have high cholesterol levels because of a condition called familial hyperlipidaemia. Your doctor can advise you if this applies to you.

● Eating oily fish regularly is a great cholesterol buster. It provides the richest source of omega-3 fats, which help to reduce triglyceride levels (another fatty substance – high triglyceride levels lead to a greater risk of cardiovascular disease).

● Foods that are high in soluble fibre can help to lower your cholesterol. Think pulses, lentils, nuts and fibre-rich fruit and veg.

● Being physically active also helps to raise your levels of 'good' HDL cholesterol.

to relax. Plus they decrease 'bad' LDL cholesterol levels. Not only that, but American researchers reported that three glasses of cranberry juice a day can raise 'good' HDL cholesterol levels by up to 10 per cent.

● **Eat a grapefruit every other day.** Grapefruits are particularly high in pectin, a soluble fibre that can help to reduce cholesterol levels. Grapefruits interfere with the absorption and processing in the liver of several medicines, however, so check with your doctor first. Other good sources of pectin include apples and berries.

● **Pour soya milk over your morning cereal.** A Spanish study of 40 men and women found that those who drank about 2 cups of soya milk a day for three months reduced their harmful LDL cholesterol levels, while at the same time increasing their beneficial HDL levels. Just make sure that you buy soya milk fortified with calcium.

● **Whip up some guacamole this evening.** Several studies find that eating one avocado a day as part of a healthy diet can lower your LDL by as much as 17 per cent while raising your HDL.

● **Spend 10 minutes a day doing strength-training exercises.** You don't have to do these at a gym – push-ups, squats, leg lifts, hip extensions – they all count. And they matter when it comes to counting your cholesterol levels: a study in the *British Journal of Sports Medicine* found that strength training lowered total cholesterol by 10 per cent and LDL cholesterol by 14 per cent among women who worked out for 45 to 50 minutes three times a week. If you can't manage that amount, start with 10 minutes a day, six days a week, and gradually work up.

● **Drink a glass of purple grape juice every day.** Rich in cholesterol-lowering flavonoids, grape juice is an extremely healthy drink, and an excellent alternative if you don't like red wine.

Whip up some guacamole.
One avocado a day can lower your LDL.

Lowering BLOOD PRESSURE

You can't see it, you can't feel it and, unless you get it checked, you won't even know you have it. That makes high blood pressure, or hypertension, a quiet killer, one that slowly damages your blood vessels, heart and eyes while simultaneously increasing your risk of heart disease, stroke, dementia and kidney disease.

As many as 45 per cent of UK adults have diagnosed high blood pressure and many more cases may be undiagnosed. The following tips will help to lower high blood pressure, or keep it from rising if it's at a healthy level. In addition, see 'Cutting back on salt', page 110, to see how reducing your salt intake can also make a difference.

18 WAYS TO GO BEYOND LOW-SALT

Choosing a home BLOOD PRESSURE MONITOR

If you decide to monitor your blood pressure at home, you will need to get a home blood pressure monitor. But there's a wide range available, so how do you know which is the best? The Blood Pressure Association in the UK advises that the easiest to use is one that is fully automatic. It also recommends that you opt for a monitor that measures your blood pressure at your upper arm rather than at your wrist or finger in order to get the most accurate results. Here's some advice about other features to look for in a home blood pressure monitor:

● Get the right size of cuff. The reading will be wrong if the cuff is the wrong size. For advice on the right size of cuff for you, go to www.bpassoc.org.uk.

● Select a monitor that has been clinically validated by the British Hypertension Society. This will ensure that it has been thoroughly tested.

● Choose a monitor you can afford. Monitors vary in price, from about £25 to over £150, and some of the more expensive models may include features that you don't need.

● Keep your monitor calibrated to make sure the reading is accurate. Send it back to the manufacturer (you may need to pay) every two years to be re-calibrated.

☺ **Eat a handful of dried apricots every afternoon.** Like bananas, apricots are a particularly good source of potassium. Plus they have lots of fibre, iron and beta carotene. The drying process actually increases the concentration of these nutrients, which are all good for your circulatory system. And as a snack, dried apricots are low in calories: roughly eight total just 100kcal. Look out for an unsulphured brand.

● **Park in the Outer Mongolia of the car park.** All you need is an extra 4,000 to 5,000 steps a day and you could lower your blood pressure by 11 points. That's what US researchers found when they tracked postmenopausal women.

● **Hold hands with your partner for 10 minutes.** That (plus a brief hug) is all it took in one study to keep blood pressure steady during a stressful incident.

● **Sleep with earplugs in tonight.** Studies suggest that being exposed to noise while you're sleeping may increase your blood pressure as well as your heart rate, so block out any noise.

● **Drink a glass of orange juice every morning and another at night.** One US study found that this lowered systolic blood pressure by an average of 7 per cent and diastolic blood pressure by an average of 4.6 per cent – thanks to the high levels of potassium in orange juice.

● **Think about your sleep.** Are you waking up tired? Is your partner complaining that you snore a lot? Talk to your doctor. You may have sleep apnoea. Studies find that half the people who have the condition, in which you stop breathing dozens or hundreds of times during the night, also have hypertension.

● **Find (and eliminate) at least one hidden source of salt a day.** For instance, did you know that many breakfast cereals contain salt? Who needs salt in their cereal? Find a brand that's salt-free.

☆ **Spend 5 minutes a day sitting in a quiet room repeating this mantra,** 'One day at a time'. Numerous studies show that meditation eases stress and lowers blood pressure. Other good mantras include: 'This, too, shall pass', 'Breathe' and 'Calm, calm, calm'.

● **Take these supplements daily:** garlic, fish oil, calcium, CoQ10. All have blood-pressure-lowering properties. Just check with your doctor first.

Stabilising your
BLOOD SUGAR

Blood sugar, or glucose, has become one of today's most studied and discussed health topics. One important reason is that diabetes, a disease reaching epidemic proportions, is directly associated with blood sugar levels. Recent research has also linked blood sugar to heart disease, memory difficulties and even fertility problems.

Whether you already have diabetes, are overweight or want to prevent future problems, here are 19 health-boosting ways to make sure your blood sugar and insulin levels are as healthy as can be. In addition, look at 'Cutting down on sugar', starting on page 101, for more ideas on stabilising your blood sugar counts.

19 TIPS FOR STABLE, STEADY GLUCOSE LEVELS

Cut carbs or cut fat?
ANSWER: **NEITHER.**

It's more important to make sure you choose the right carbs and the right fats. Carbs from sugary foods and white breads and pasta raise blood sugar, while 'good' carbs – whole grains, fruit, vegetables, beans, lentils, nuts and seeds – help to stabilise it. Similarly, some fats – the saturated fats in meats and full-fat dairy and trans fats such as hydrogenated oils – are bad for your health, while the polyunsaturated and monounsaturated oils in nuts, seeds, olives, avocados and fish reduce the risk of diabetes.

8 hours. Numerous studies find that sleep deprivation has a dramatic effect on your blood sugar and insulin levels. If you need help falling (and staying) asleep, see 'The Sleep Routine', on page 72, for tips on getting a better rest.

☻ **Ask your partner if you snore.** Harvard researchers found that women who snored were more than twice as likely as those who didn't to develop diabetes – regardless of weight, smoking history or family history of diabetes. If you do snore, see your doctor. You may have a physical problem, or you may simply need to lose some weight and change the way you sleep.

Eat soba noodles for dinner one night a week. They are an excellent source of fibre.

☻ Prepare your breakfast, lunch and dinner, but then divide each meal in half. Eat half now, then the other half in a couple of hours. Eating several small meals rather than three large meals helps to avoid the major influx of glucose that, in turn, results in a blood sugar surge and a big release of insulin.

☻ **Don't skip a meal.** Your blood sugar drops like a rock when you're starving (hence the headache and shakiness). Then when you do eat, you flood your system with glucose, forcing your pancreas to release more insulin and creating a dangerous cycle.

☻ **Go to bed at 10pm, wake up at 6am.** Adjust the hours accordingly so that you're always getting a consistent

☻ **Spend 10 minutes a day tensing then relaxing each muscle in your body,** from your toes to your eyes. The technique is called progressive muscle relaxation, and a study of 100 people with high blood sugar levels found that this kind of stress-relief significantly improved their blood sugar levels. For other tips, see 'Defusing Stress', on page 270.

☻ **Eat 75g of beans a day.** These high-fibre foods take longer to digest, so they release their glucose more slowly. Studies find just 75g a day can help to stabilise blood sugar and insulin levels.

☺ **Sprinkle a few walnuts over your salad.** Walnuts are great sources of monounsaturated fat, which won't raise your blood sugar as many other foods do. And some researchers suspect that this fat even makes cells more sensitive to insulin, helping to combat high blood sugar.

Preventing **CANCER**

Consider this number: 10 million. That's how many cases of cancer are diagnosed worldwide each year. Now consider this number: 15 million. That's how many cases of cancer the World Health Organisation estimates will be diagnosed in the year 2020 – a 50 per cent increase – if we don't take some preventive action.

The truth is, most cancers don't develop overnight or out of nowhere. Cancer is largely predictable, the end result of a decades-long process, rather like heart disease. And, like heart disease, just a few health-boosting changes in your daily life can significantly reduce your risk of developing the dreaded 'Big C'. Here are 27 of the best pieces of advice.

27 WAYS TO HELP PROTECT YOURSELF AGAINST THE BIG C

Greater
LUNG POWER

If you want to be able to blow out all the candles on your cake when you're 75 (assuming your family dares to put on a candle for every year), not to mention climb three flights of stairs without needing oxygen, now is the time to take action. What, you're wondering, could you possibly do beyond quitting smoking to get your bellows in better shape? The answer: plenty. Although stopping smoking is at the top of any list, here are another 15 tips that will have you doing less huffing and puffing, as well as protecting your lungs from damage and disease. In addition, read about proper breathing technique on page 273, part of the discussion on managing stress.

15 WAYS TO BREATHE EASIER

Have a heart-to-heart with your sleeping partner. The key question to ask: do I snore? If the answer is yes, make an appointment with your GP and ask for a referral to a sleep centre to get checked for sleep apnoea. This condition, in which someone stops breathing dozens or even hundreds of times during the night, can actually damage the lungs nearly as much as smoking. Fortunately, it's treatable.

 Make several trips up and down stairs every day. The kind of exercise that makes your heart beat faster, such as climbing stairs, riding a bike or walking briskly, is very important for keeping your heart and lungs in good shape. For instance, studies find that walking for about 15 minutes at a time, three to four times a day, improved breathing in people with the lung disease emphysema.

 Make sure you get enough omega-3. Most airway problems, including asthma, are related to inflammation. Omega-3 fatty acids reduce inflammation.

 Breathe from your abdomen for at least 5 minutes every day. This kind of breathing, called diaphragmatic breathing, involves training and strengthening your diaphragm so that it requires less effort to take in each breath. To do it, inhale deeply through your nose, filling your lungs from the bottom up. If you're doing it right, your stomach will push out. Exhale and repeat.

 Expand your chest like a cocky rooster. To help your chest to expand and boost your lung capacity, lie on your back with your knees bent and your feet flat on the floor. Place your hands behind your head and bring your elbows together so they're nearly touching. As you inhale, let your elbows drop to the sides slowly so your arms are flat on the floor when your lungs are full. As you exhale, raise your elbows again.

 Make spaghetti sauce tonight, tomato and basil salad tomorrow night and roast tomatoes over the weekend. British researchers found that people who ate tomatoes three times a week had improved lung function and experienced less wheeziness and fewer asthma-like symptoms.

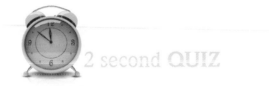

2 second **QUIZ**

Apple or orange?
ANSWER: **APPLE.**

The old adage is true after all. A study from the University of Nottingham found that people who ate more than five apples a week had improved lung function, less wheeziness and fewer asthma-like symptoms. Eat them raw, try them baked, add them diced into a salad or sauté an apple with onions as a side dish for chicken or fish.

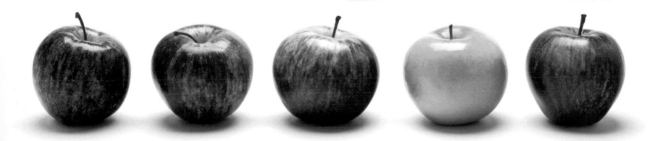

● **Read the fine print on household cleaners.** Some products, such as oven cleaner, can be toxic if inhaled. If the instructions say to open a window or use in a well-ventilated space, make sure you do so. And wear a face mask when working around toxic dust or fumes. Even simple household tasks such as sanding paint could send damaging fragments into your lungs.

● **Work in 10 to 20 crunches a day.** Your abdominal and chest muscles allow you to suck air in and out. Strengthen them, as well as practising your deep breathing, to get the breathing power of a professional opera singer (or at least close).

● **Take your medicine and listen to your doctor if you have asthma.** There's some good evidence that people with asthma eventually develop chronic obstructive pulmonary disease, or COPD, a lung disease that strikes people aged 65 and older. There's also evidence that keeping your asthma under control can prevent the disease from developing.

● **Look on the bright side.** When Harvard researchers followed 670 men with an average age of 63 for eight years,

they found that the optimists had much better lung function and a slower rate of lung function decline than the pessimists.

☆ **Get at least seven servings of fruit and vegetables a day.** A 1998 study found that the high amounts of antioxidants they contain, including vitamin C, vitamin E, selenium and beta carotene, meant better lung function – even in smokers.

● **Have a glass of wine tonight.** Drinking wine, particularly white wine, both in the recent past and over your lifetime, seems to help your lungs, possibly because of wine's high antioxidant levels. It has to be wine, though; researchers found no such correlation when they looked at the effects of other forms of alcohol.

☆ **Brush your teeth twice a day and floss after every meal.** American researchers found that patients with periodontal – gum – disease were 1½ times more likely also to have COPD. The worse the gum disease, the worse the lung function, suggesting a direct correlation between the two.

● **Say no to dessert.** A 2004 study has revealed that carrying extra weight makes your respiratory muscles work harder and less efficiently. This results in shortness of breath, making it hard to exercise, which makes it hard to lose the weight ... To break out of this depressing cycle follow the tips in 'Losing Weight', page 199.

● **In hot, dry or very cold weather, or in dusty or polluted air,** breathe in through your nose and out through your mouth. Our nasal passages are designed to filter the air and regulate its temperature and humidity. If you breathe in through your mouth, everything – dust, coldness, etc. – goes straight on into the lungs.

Flossing helps
to protect
lung health.

Greater **MOBILITY**

If you've ever crawled out of bed in the morning aching as if you'd played a mean game of rugby in your sleep, heard your knees creaking as you descended the stairs or needed two ibuprofen before you could even bend over to tie your shoelaces, then this chapter is for you.

Making some simple changes to your diet and daily activities – even just to the way you sit – coupled with taking a few key supplements a day, can save a lot of wear and tear on your joints and ligaments as well as reduce your pain. Here are the top tips to help you where you hurt.

17 WAYS TO KEEP YOUR JOINTS AGILE AND ARTHRITIS AT BAY

Do **THREE** things…

If you do only three things for back pain, doctors concur that these make the most sense:

1 Get up and go. The old idea of lying around when your back hurts just makes things worse. As soon as the acute stage of back pain is over, you need to get up and move. Walking is great. So are stretching exercises.

2 Make sure you're sleeping on the right mattress. One study of 313 men with lower back pain found that those who slept on a medium-firm mattress were twice as likely to get some pain relief. If your mattress is more than ten years old, it's time to go mattress shopping.

3 Wear soft-soled shoes with low heels. High heels throw your entire body out of alignment, contributing not only to back pain but also to knee and hip pain and injuries as well, not to mention what they do to your feet.

effective and low-cost way of rehabilitating the hand and wrist after injury or surgery. It will also keep your wrists and hands flexible with good blood circulation if you have arthritis or other painful problems.

● **Enhance the range of motion in your wrist with this exercise.** Slowly bend your wrist backwards and forwards, holding for a 5 second count in each position. Do three sets – ten times for each hand – twice a day.

● **Always bend from the knees, not the back, when lifting.** Also, keep the weight you're carrying close to your body, as if carrying a baby, for less risk of back strain.

● **Crunch your way through 20 modified sit-ups every morning.** These strengthen the abdominal muscles while stretching and relaxing the back. To do a modified sit-up, bend your knees or place your feet on a small stool or chair as you complete the crunch.

▐▐▐▶ **On long drives, take a break every hour,** get out of the car and walk around for 5 minutes, stretching like a cat. Your back will thank you later.

● **For back relief, get on your hands and knees** (on a padded surface) and round your back, again like a scared cat. Hold for 5 seconds, then let your stomach relax and sag for 5 seconds. Do two sets of ten each any time you've been sitting for more than an hour.

● **Serve up some pickled herring for lunch or supper.** It's rich in omega-3 fatty acids, shown to reduce inflammation and alleviate pain from arthritis.

● **Play a computer game, read a book or watch a film when your joints are hurting.** Researchers find that concentrating on what you're doing distracts you from your pain.

● **Quit smoking.** Smoking narrows the arteries and reduces your circulation and that, according to a study in the medical journal *Spine*, increases your risk of back pain and slows healing.

Smoking ups your risk of back pain.

Stronger **BONES**

Drink your milk! Surely you remember your mother admonishing you with those very words when you were a child. And she was right: children who drink plenty of milk (or who get plenty of calcium from other sources) grow up to have less risk of osteoporosis, the disease that causes bones to become thin and brittle. It appears that many of us didn't take the advice, though; annually, osteoporosis accounts for about 230,000 fractures in the UK. One in two British women and one in five British men over the age of 50 will break a bone, mainly because of poor bone health. Yet even as an adult there's plenty you can do to protect yourself, from increasing your calcium intake to getting the right exercise. Pay special attention to this advice if you're over 50, have a family history of osteoporosis or are a woman who has gone through menopause, because your bones may be more vulnerable.

20 WAYS TO HELP TO PREVENT OSTEOPOROSIS

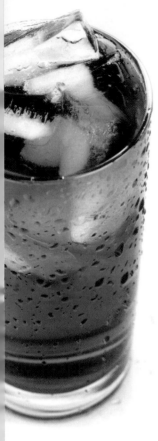

Choose delicious iced tea or water, not fizzy drinks.

● **Have a pizza topped with sardines and spinach.** Not only is it delicious (go on, give it a try), but you'll get bone-protecting calcium in every bite.

● **Have four dried figs for a midafternoon snack.** Dried figs are a great source of calcium. Sprinkle a few diced figs over your yoghurt and you'll meet more than half your daily calcium needs (four dried figs, about 60g, contain almost a fifth – 17 per cent – of your RDA).

● **Sip water or iced tea instead of fizzy drinks.** An American study found that women who drank at least one 330ml can of cola every day for four years had up to 5 per cent lower bone mineral density than women who drank fewer than one a week. All the women were drinking the same amount of milk, so researchers think the phosphoric acid in fizzy drinks affects the body's absorption of calcium.

● **Hang room-darkening shades in your bedroom.** You'll sleep much better without ambient light, and sleep is important for bone. Much of your bone remodelling, in which old bone is replaced by new, occurs during sleep. If you're not sleeping enough, when do you think your body is going to perform this valuable job?

☆ **Walk for 30 minutes a day.** Most women lose 3 to 6 per cent of their bone mass every year during the five years before and after menopause. But women who walked regularly (about 7.5 miles a week) took four to seven years longer to lose the same amount of bone as women who didn't walk at all. Walking briskly, you should be able to cover 2 miles in 30 minutes; walk for 30 minutes just four days a week and you'll get the 7.5 miles in. Add an extra day, just for good measure.

☆ **Start a vegetable and flower garden.** US researchers found that gardening (and weight training) were strongly associated with reducing the risk of osteoporosis in 3,310 women aged 50 and older. It turns out that pushing a lawnmower, thrusting a shovel into the ground, lifting heavy wheelbarrows filled with mulch, raking, carrying and pulling weeds are all great weight-bearing exercises. Would you rather lift weights in a sweaty gym or plant and harvest your own ruby-red tomatoes?

● **Sign up for a tai chi class at your local community hall or sports centre.** Several studies have found that tai chi cut the risk of falling by nearly a half and reduced the rate of fractures even in people who had falls. Ideally, you should practise tai chi for 10 to 15 minutes at a time, once or twice a week, to gain the benefits.

● **Make a pot of low-fat yoghurt a daily snack.** With 210mg of calcium in a small pot (150ml) of low-fat yoghurt, you're a quarter of the way to your RDA.

● **Swap peas for frozen fresh soyabeans this evening.** The science is still evolving, but it seems that the natural plant oestrogens in soya help to strengthen bone in the same way that our own hormones do.

2 second QUIZ

Swimming or walking
ANSWER: **WALKING.**

While swimming is a great exercise for your lungs and heart, it doesn't do anything for your bones, because there's little resistance in water.

STRONGER LIBIDO, better sex

Your parents probably never told you this, but it's true: sex is good for you! Plenty of studies show it: regular sex increases immunity from viruses, relieves stress and even helps to protect the health of a man's prostate gland by emptying the fluids held there. It also triggers the release of chemicals that improve mood and ease pain. While menopause in women does affect sexual drive and function somewhat, there is no reason why healthy men and women can't experience sexual pleasure throughout their lives. The nature and intensity of the sex may change, but the love and pleasure don't. So if your sex drive has stalled, try a couple of health-boosting tips to get your engine ticking over again in no time.

26 WAYS TO GET THERE

2 second QUIZ

Cream cake or an orange
ANSWER: **ORANGE.**

A US study of 32 obese women found that more than half of those who lost weight said their sex lives improved.

Lose weight for more vitality.

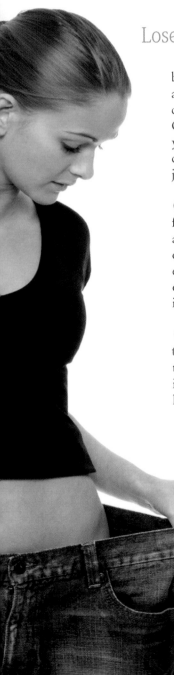

bath ready in the evening? How about a meal out every Tuesday – when most couples are slumped in front of the TV? Or massaging your partner's feet while you watch a DVD together? The key is consistency. These are not things you do just once, but over and over again.

● **Get a massage.** Or a pedicure, or a facial, or whatever makes you feel better about yourself. If you take care of your own body, you're much more likely to enjoy it. Another good way to take care of yourself is to exercise. An extra benefit is better blood flow to crucial organs.

● **Turn the timer on for 15 minutes and talk to him (or her)** about anything other than children, money problems or work issues. Talk about the dream you had last night, an article you read, the great presentation you made. When the timer goes off, it's your partner's turn.

● **Go away for a couple of days – by yourself.** While you're away, make a list of all the things you love and like about your partner. Close your eyes and picture yourself making love.

Call him or her and have an erotic phone conversation. By the time you get home, you'll be greedy for each other.

● **Send the children away and stay at home together.** Make love in a different part of the house, be it your bath or a blanket in front of the fireplace.

● **Before you go to bed, take a few minutes** to write out a to-do list and a list of your worries. This gets rid of the anxieties that can often interfere with your ability to relax and become aroused.

● **Spend an hour touching every part of your partner's body – without using your hands.** Use other parts of your body instead. Conversely, caress one another, with your hands touching every part of the body except the genital zones. This can remove any pressure you might feel to 'get right to it' after a hectic day and is a wonderful way to relax and escape from the daily grind and transition from other (oh-so-non-sexual) roles.

● **Stop at one (or two) drinks.** A small amount of alcohol can set the mood; more can drown the flame of desire, or lessen your ability to see your desire through.

● **Create a romantic CD.** Have it playing when your partner returns home. Light a few scented candles while you're at it.

☺ **Tell your partner two things you love about him or her every day.** Love, affection and mutual respect are the bases for a steamy sex life.

● **Do something physical together,** for example, skiing, a long country walk, a stroll along a beach, canoeing. Such activities create a sense of physical vitality that readily translates into intimacy.

Combating
ALLERGIES

If the constant drip, sniff, sneeze and itch of allergies make you think of buying shares in the company that makes Kleenex, dry your eyes and prepare to take action. You're going to wage battle inside your house and even inside your body to reduce the number of allergy attacks you suffer and minimise those annoying symptoms. Allergies may not be life-threatening, but they're nothing to sneeze at either. Here are 16 of the best ways to protect yourself. Plus, turn to 'The cleaning routine', on page 68, for more on safe, healthy ways to purge your home of allergens.

16 WAYS TO STOP BEING SNEEZY

Improving your **VISION**

Chances are you take your eyes for granted. Most of us do. So imagine if you couldn't gaze at your family or even navigate your way safely round the kitchen. Research by the College of Optometrists in the UK estimates that 65 per cent of British people could be at risk of future eyesight problems because of their diet. A well-balanced diet can protect against age-related macular degeneration (AMD), which affects roughly 500,000 people in the UK and is the leading cause of blindness in people over 50 in the Western world. The good news: the most common diseases are all preventable to some extent. The first step, if you smoke, is to stop. Smoking increases your risk of major eye conditions.

21 WAYS TO SEE CLEARLY FOR EVER

Mix a handful of blueberries with a cup of yoghurt for breakfast this morning. Blueberries are one of the richest fruit forms of antioxidants. A study published in *The Archives of Ophthalmology* found that women and men who ate the greatest amount of fruit were the least likely to develop age-related macular degeneration (AMD), the leading cause of blindness in older people.

Have spinach or kale twice a week. It could be a spinach quiche, steamed kale or maybe Tuscan spinach – sautéed in some olive oil with garlic and raisins. Regardless, be sure to get as much of both as you can. Studies find that lutein, a nutrient that is particularly abundant in spinach and kale, may prevent age-related macular degeneration and cataracts (AMD). Ideally, get your lutein in combination with some form of fat (olive oil works well) for the best absorption.

● Cook with red onions, not white. Red onions contain far more quercetin, an antioxidant that is thought to protect against cataracts.

● Aim your car vents at your feet – not your eyes. Dry, air-conditioned air will suck the moisture out of the eyes. Aim the vents in your car away from your eyes, or wear sunglasses as a shield. Dry eyes can be more than an inconvenience; serious dryness can lead to corneal abrasions and even blindness if left untreated.

● Walk at least four times a week. Some evidence suggests that regular exercise can reduce the intraocular pressure, or IOP, in people with glaucoma. In one study, glaucoma patients who walked briskly four times a week for 40 minutes lowered their IOP enough for them to stop taking medication for the condition.

Healthy **INVESTMENT**

Sunglasses
Make sure they're close-fitting, preferably wraparound, and block out 99 to 100 per cent of UVA and UVB rays. Step outside while wearing them before you buy to make sure they do a good job of blocking glare and yet aren't too dark.

Move your computer screen to just below eye level. Your eyes will close slightly when you're staring at the computer, minimising fluid evaporation and the risk of a condition called dry eye syndrome.

● Twice a week, walk away from greasy or sweet snacks. A 2001 study found that people whose diets were high in omega-3 fatty acids and low in omega-6 fatty acids (found in many fat-filled snack foods such as pre-prepared pies, cakes, biscuits and crisps) were significantly less likely to develop AMD

Red onions may keep cataracts at bay.

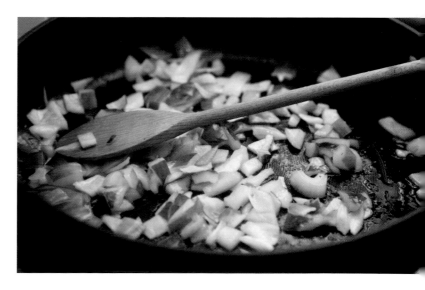

How loud **IS TOO LOUD?**

Exposure of just 1 minute to sounds of 110 decibels or higher can damage your hearing.
No more than 15 minutes of unprotected exposure is recommended for noises of 100 decibels, as well as several hours' exposure to noises of 90 decibels or higher. Here's the decibel level of some common noises:

- **140 decibels:**   rock concerts, fireworks
- **110 decibels:**   chainsaw
- **100 decibels:**   woodworking equipment
- **90 decibels:**   lawnmower, motorcycle
- **80 decibels:**   city traffic noise
- **60 decibels:**   normal conversation
- **40 decibels:**   refrigerator humming
- **20 decibels:**   whispered voice
- **0 decibels:**   threshold of normal hearing

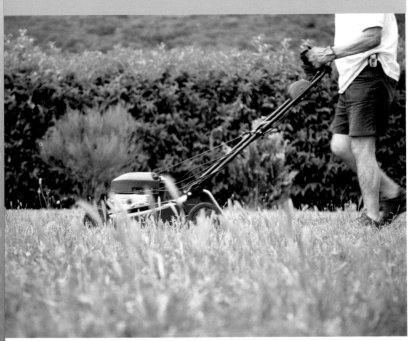

● **Get five servings of veg a day.** When researchers explored the connection between a variety of lifestyle factors and sudden deafness in 109 patients, comparing their deaf patients to those with normal hearing, they found that those who ate the most fresh veg had the lowest risk of sudden deafness. See page 83 for ways to sneak veg into your diet.

☺ **Ask your doctor to clear the wax from your ears.** It's often all that's needed to improve your hearing. Just don't try it yourself; sticking pointed objects into your ear canal is a no-no. If you want to de-wax at home, try wax-softening ear drops, sold at chemists. If the wax doesn't liquefy and find its way out, see your GP's practice nurse to request ear syringeing.

● **Go to bed and rest when you have a cold.** That gives your body the strength to fight off the infection and reduces the risk that it will develop into something more serious, such as an ear infection, which could eventually affect your hearing.

● **Make earplugs a standard part of your wardrobe.** Keep a pair in your bag, in your car, in the garage with the gardening tools and by the lawnmower. That way, if you find yourself unable to escape from loud noise, you're always prepared to protect your hearing.

● **Get a friend to stand next to you while you're plugged into your iPod** (or MP3 player). If your friend can hear it through your earphones, it's too loud.

● **Try a ginkgo biloba supplement.** Some studies suggest that the herb might not only help with ringing in the ears (tinnitus), but may also benefit hearing loss by improving blood flow to the ears. The herb takes weeks to work, so be patient.

Sharpen your senses of **SMELL & TASTE**

We all know that feeling of having a bad taste in the mouth, or the way a stuffy nose makes even the most fragrant garlic pizza taste like cardboard. But did you know that your senses of smell and taste naturally decline as you age? Often the change is so gradual that you barely notice it. That wouldn't be a problem, except that it can affect your health – studies find that people with an impaired ability to smell and taste tend to follow less healthy diets. It also puts you in danger: your sense of smell serves as an early-warning system for things like rotten food and gas leaks.

Here's how to sustain your senses of smell and taste so that every bite (and sniff) tells you what you need to know.

19 SENSIBLE STRATEGIES

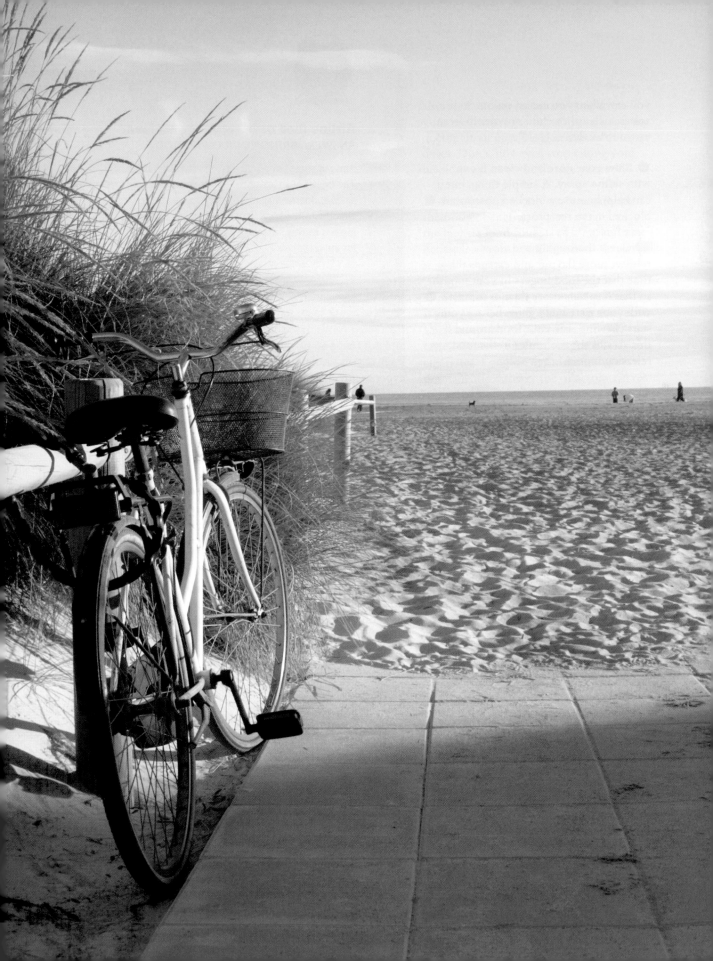

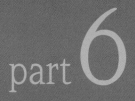

part 6

MENTAL RELIEF

Attitudes can harm, and attitudes can heal – science has proved both beyond question. For better health, here's how to replace stress and worry with calm and happiness.

Defusing **STRESS**

Some days it seems as if life throws stress at you from all directions.
It can drain your energy, destroy your good mood and challenge your outlook. But science has shown that stress also causes your body to release hormones that raise blood pressure, speed up your heart and breathing, halt digestion, cause a surge in blood sugar and more. When stress is ongoing, this constant physical reaction can significantly raise your risk of colds, diabetes, heart disease, back troubles and almost every other major health concern. Yet stress can be relatively easy to manage. All it takes is mental commitment – and an open mind. So give some of these health-boosting approaches to stress management a try.

34 WAYS TO CALM YOURSELF DOWN

Embrace the number one truth about stress: only you create it. Stress isn't defined as a large workload, a difficult child or a rise in terrorism. Stress is your physical and mental reaction to these external stimuli. Consider the saying about alcoholism – that admitting to being an alcoholic is more than 50 per cent of the cure. The same is true for stress: embracing the fact that stress is your reaction to external stimuli – and not the stimuli themselves – is half the battle towards managing it. You can't change a crazy world. But you can learn to handle it with humour, humility and hope. So it should come as no surprise that virtually every stress-relief method that follows is about how to improve your reaction to external factors.

● **Give your partner a hug every day before work.** It's so simple, yet so often overlooked when you're trying to make your lunch, find your shoes and keys and get on the road before rush hour. American researchers discovered that the few seconds it takes to hug your partner can help you to remain calm as chaos unfolds around you.

● **Buy yourself flowers once a week and display them prominently on your desk.** Women who sat near a bouquet of flowers were found to be more relaxed during a typing assignment than women who didn't have flowers, according to a US study.

● **Take a deep breath, then try to see yourself in someone else's shoes.** Consider for a minute that your boss and others who annoy you may be experiencing just as much inner turmoil as they are creating around them. When people are rude, they are often suffering in one way or another.

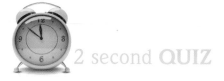

Needlework or cooking?
ANSWER: **NEEDLEWORK.**

At least for most people. Research shows that repetitive tasks such as embroidery and crochet can reduce stress just as effectively as meditation or yoga. Many people find cooking relaxing, but unless you are preparing a very familiar dish with no margin for error, it does take mental energy and it can be stressful.

● **See the time waiting in a queue as a chance to relax.** When you make a split decision about which queue to join at the supermarket, chances are some other queue will move more quickly. In a worst-case scenario, a customer in front of you has to have the price of one or more items checked by an assistant who takes for ever to get back. Rather than sending your stress hormones into the stratosphere as you steam over your bad luck, think about how busy you usually are and recognise this – in reality, usually just a few minutes – as a gift, as a time when you can just relax. As you wait, think about the things in life for which you are grateful, meditate on your breath, talk to one of the other customers or look at a magazine.

▐▐▐▶ **Develop a ritual in the morning** that focuses on calmness, beauty and the people who support you, or anything that helps you to feel a sense of peace. You might, for example, spend a few moments reminding yourself of your blessings. Your ritual might involve sitting outside (weather permitting), taking in your surroundings and appreciating the sounds of the birds and the sights of the sun glistening off the leaves and grass. If

Defusing **ANGER**

Furious. Annoyed. Enraged. Outraged. Irate. Maddened. Raging. Riled. Wrathful. All synonyms for one of the most common human emotions: anger. There's no way to get through life without getting angry. The key is to learn how to defuse that anger constructively so that it doesn't end up destroying your health. Bottling up anger can increase your levels of homocysteine, a chemical linked to heart disease. It can also raise your cholesterol levels and heart rate, suppress your immune system, lead to depression and even give you a heart attack. But by defusing your anger you can reduce your risk of these health conditions. Here's how to let off steam safely and protect your health.

24 WAYS TO RELEASE YOUR EMOTIONAL STEAM

● **If you are angry with a politician, policy or some public injustice, do something about it.** In one American study, researchers tracked the brain-wave patterns of students who had just been told the university was considering big tuition increases. They all exhibited brain patterns signifying anger, but signing a petition to block the increases seemed to provide satisfaction. Put simply, working to right a wrong is life-affirming and positive. Stewing in a bad situation without taking action has the opposite result.

● **Forget about punching a pillow, a wall or the object of your anger.** Contrary to popular belief, these common reactions don't decrease your anger. In fact, studies find, they only increase your hostility.

▶ **Take three deep breaths.** When you're angry, your body becomes tense. Breathing deeply helps to lower your internal anger meter.

● **Know why you feel angry.** Think like a detective and track down clues about the kinds of situations, people and events that trigger your anger. Once you're aware of them, try to avoid them if possible. If you can't avoid them, at least you'll know to anticipate them, which will give you more time to prepare for them so that they don't affect you so negatively.

☺ **Keep in mind that whoever loses it, loses.** Losing your temper makes you look like the bad guy to everyone else, no matter who is really at fault. To get better at controlling your anger, visualise a scene in which you got angry and replay the tape several times, each time imagining yourself responding in a different way. You're actually rehearsing different reactions and giving yourself new

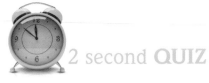

2 second QUIZ

Hold in anger or express it?
ANSWER: **EXPRESS YOUR ANGER.**

The real damage of a type A personality (see page 279) doesn't come from ambition, but from repressed anger. If you're angry, get it under control, then express it. But don't fixate on the anger; instead, concentrate on the underlying causes and issues. Try to be fair, but also be honest.

options. The next time you're close to losing your temper, one of these options will pop into your mind, providing you with a better response.

● **Picture a red stop sign in your mind** or wear a rubber band on your wrist and snap it whenever you find your anger beginning to boil. Then take a few minutes to put the issue into perspective and ask yourself if it's worth the humiliation that comes from becoming overtly angry.

● **Recognise your own personal signs of escalating anger.** These might be clenched fists, trembling, flushing, sweating. Then use deep breathing to regain control of yourself before your anger erupts. If you're not sure about your own anger warning signs, ask a friend or family member. It's pretty likely they'll know!

☆ **Pinch yourself every time you hear yourself using the words 'never', 'always', etc.** Such thinking leads to a black-and-white, all-or-nothing mentality and that, in turn, shortens your fuse. Instead, look at things in shades of grey. Acknowledge that life can be unfair and that sometimes people do the wrong

Plane, car or train?
ANSWER: **CAR OR TRAIN.**

Flying might seem to be the fastest option but, if your destination is less than 300 miles away, just think of the time spent driving to an airport, parking, getting through security and boarding – not to mention delays and even overbooked flights. So catch a train, if it's convenient, or drive. A direct train can be very relaxing, especially if you don't need transport at the other end. But in a car, you have more control over the situation, you're in your own environment and, if you check the traffic situation first and adjust your route accordingly, fewer things can go wrong (such as hold-ups and cancellations).

● Most people aren't very good judges of how their actions affect others. In other words, we're neither villains nor saints. We're all just people – struggling to lead happy, healthy, meaningful lives in a complicated world. Yes, even the people who anger you. With this in mind, forgiveness comes much easier.

▐▐▐▶ **Get angry with the person who can make a difference.** There's nothing to be gained by becoming angry with the poor soul who is simply caught in the crossfire. This advice is particularly important when you're dealing with people who work in the service industries. Is it the fault of the salesperson that something you need is out of stock? No, but his or her manager could probably fix things.

● **Understand that someone, somewhere,** is gossiping about you, because that's what people do, but understand also that it has absolutely no impact on your life.

● **Take responsibility for your anger.** Recognise that it's your choice whether or not you become angry.

● **Talk about your anger.** This is different from expressing it; talking about it means unloading and decompressing with a friend, going over the situation with a neutral observer who can bring some perspective to the situation, or even talking out loud to yourself about it (preferably when no one else can hear you).

● **Get on your bike and go for a half-hour ride.** Or jump up and down on a trampoline. Or go for a vigorous swim. Or attack the weeds in your garden. Any kind of vigorous, intense physical activity helps to dissipate anger.

● **Get some perspective.** Is this person or situation really worth spending your emotional energy on? Risking your health over? Putting your dignity and peace of mind at risk?

If you want to lose your anger, get on your bike.

Dealing with
ANXIETY

You know the feeling. You're doing fine, then your son announces that he's dropping out of university, and you discover you need a new roof. Suddenly, you can't breathe. Your chest hurts and you're convinced it's a heart attack. It's more likely you're having an anxiety attack — an acute reaction to intense stress. According to the Office of National Statistics in the UK, an estimated 4.7 per cent of adults experience generalised anxiety disorders, not including depression, at any one time; it is also thought that 7 people in every 1,000 will develop a panic disorder. Sometimes medication and therapy are needed, but quite often learning to cope when anxiety hits can make a big difference. Here are 17 ways to do it.

17 WAYS TO STOP WORRYING

Laugh or cry?
ANSWER: **CRY.**

When life is so challenging that you're having anxiety attacks, it's a serious business. While laughing off the situation may seem like a mature, 'I'm in control' response, it may be masking or denying some very unhealthy issues. Crying is a more honest, anxiety-releasing response, with positive physiological effects. It also signals to you and your loved ones that all is not well and that change may be in order.

▶ **Name your fears.** The most anxiety-producing thing of all is the unknown. So make a point of dragging your worries out of the shadows. If you're worried about your son/daughter/partner getting hurt or killed in a car crash, for example, discuss it – at least with yourself. Look up the statistics on driving and injury to relieve your mind. Do the same for whatever else makes you worry, whether it's Ebola virus, bioterrorism, cancer or plane crashes. Once you name your fears and learn more about them, you can take steps to minimise your risk. You'll also find that the fears you name and tame are far less menacing than the fears left to lurk in the shadows of your imagination.

● **Make sure you're getting several servings of whole grains, fruit and vegetables every day,** along with healthy protein sources such as fish, poultry, lentils, soya or lean meats. The combination of healthy foods helps your brain to make serotonin, a chemical that induces a state of calm relaxation.

A good diet that includes plenty of fish and vegetables helps your brain to make serotonin, a chemical that induces relaxation.

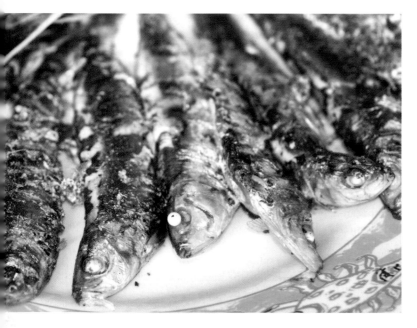

● **Go to the museum, see a film, read a good book or take up oil painting** (or some other hobby). People who are bored tend to score higher on tests designed to measure levels of anxiety.

● **Rent a meditation, tai chi or yoga DVD from the library.** They are all effective, non-medical ways of dealing with anxiety.

● **Share your anxieties with a confidant.** It's a good idea to find someone who can help you to understand why you worry too much. If appropriate, try to play the same role for that person. We are usually better at putting someone else's worries in perspective than we are our own.

DEPRESSION

There comes a point when most of us realise: life sometimes isn't much fun. It may have been an eye-opening adventure in our youth, our teens, even our 20s, but, as time passes, the glee of living gets harder to sustain. Most of us cope just fine with this. With age, exuberance and excitement get replaced by a more subtle but deeper joy. We have families and friends we love, meaningful jobs, hobbies and holidays that provide real pleasure, accumulated wisdom that gives us a sense of value. But for millions of people, the path of life occasionally leads to depression. The point here is not to give you a diagnosis or treatment – that's for professionals to do. But even if you are taking medication for depression, the following lifestyle tactics may increase the drug's effectiveness. If you're simply feeling low, the tips may give you the boost you need to pull you up without the need for prescription drugs.

16 WAYS TO BANISH THE BLUES

Dealing with **GUILT**

Ask anyone to define 'guilt', and they'll hum and haw. It's hard to describe, a feeling of 'I should have done something, should be doing something, should not have done something.' The *Oxford English Dictionary* defines it as 'a feeling of having done wrong or failed in an obligation'. It's a revealing definition – it's a *feeling* of having done wrong rather than *doing* wrong. Of course, sometimes you should feel guilty (if you've committed a crime, say, or intentionally hurt someone). But if you're like most of us, you feel guilty because of all the 'shoulds' in your life. That's bad for your mental and physical health, so read on to find out how to shed some of that guilt.

19 TIPS FOR A CLEARER CONSCIENCE

☆ **Above all else, learn to forgive yourself.** If feelings of guilt haunt you, take some concrete steps to end this self-inflicted punishment. First, list the things you feel guilty about. It could be something stupid you said recently, an act of cruelty against a sibling in your childhood or a detrimental personal habit that has hurt your relationship with a loved one. Then ask, 'How can I forgive myself and let it go?' Perhaps it's saying a prayer, writing a letter, having a talk, making a charitable donation or committing to personal change. Often it's merely having the courage to say, 'I'm sorry.' Then do what it takes so you can honestly, finally forgive yourself. You'll be amazed at the lightness this can bring.

● **Set a no-guilt-allowed rule whenever you go on holiday or do something just for yourself.** Often people, particularly women, do not experience holidays, breaks and other relaxing activities as stress-relieving because they feel guilty that they're not doing more productive things. Tell yourself that you are taking a break and doing it for a reason (improved health, decreased stress, etc.), so there is no reason to feel guilty. As soon as you hear yourself say, 'I should be …' remind yourself why you are choosing not to do that. Make sure anyone you're travelling with knows about the no-guilt rule too.

● **Take 5 minutes in the morning to feel guilty.** Then either resolve what's triggering the guilt (for example, call your mother) or forgive yourself for what you did that you shouldn't have done, knowing that you've learned your lesson and won't do it again.

▐▐▶ **Correct a mistake rather than feeling guilty about it.** For instance, if you're feeling guilty because you went shopping

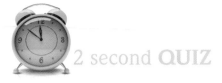

2 second QUIZ

Letter or phone call?
ANSWER: LETTER.

When an apology is due, sit down and write a letter. Not only will it give you a better opportunity to think through your thoughts, but you always have the option of sending it or not sending it. Sometimes the simple act of writing is enough to give you peace of mind. If you do send it, the person to whom you're sending it has a lifetime reminder of your apology.

on Saturday instead of going to see a relative in hospital, take time out of your schedule for a midweek visit. Many times, the things we feel guilty about are relatively easy to put right.

▐▐▶ **Recognise that a feeling of guilt doesn't always mean that what you did was wrong.** For instance, if you're feeling guilty because you decided it was more important to relax with a book than to have coffee with your always-in-a-crisis friend, that means you're learning to set limits and take time for yourself. In cases like this, have the confidence to admit that you made the right choice.

● **Commit to saying no** at least once a day – no guilt allowed.

● **Start a guilt diary.** Every time you feel guilty about something, write it down in your diary. Write the time, the day, what you feel guilty about. Go back and reread this diary every couple of weeks to find the trends in your guilt. This will provide clues to the source that will enable you to deal better with its underlying roots.

Coping with **GRIEF**

There's nothing more uncontrollable than the death of someone you love. But there are ways to cope. The following tips can help you to move through what may seem like endless grief. Note the pattern in the suggestions – maintaining your love for the person and honouring his or her memory, while still moving on with your life:

● Think of your grief as a certain number of tears you must shed before the intensity of the sadness, anger and guilt subsides. The more opportunities you take to grieve and feel all the related feelings, the sooner you will reach your magic number of tears.

● Create a special place in your house, with a picture, a candle and perhaps some small mementos of your loved one. When you feel sad, spend some time there, and 'talk' to the person you lost about how you're feeling.

● Get a scrapbook and make a memory album of the good times you had together. Put in photos, greetings cards, menus or postcards. You can also write in it. Refer back to it in times of sadness.

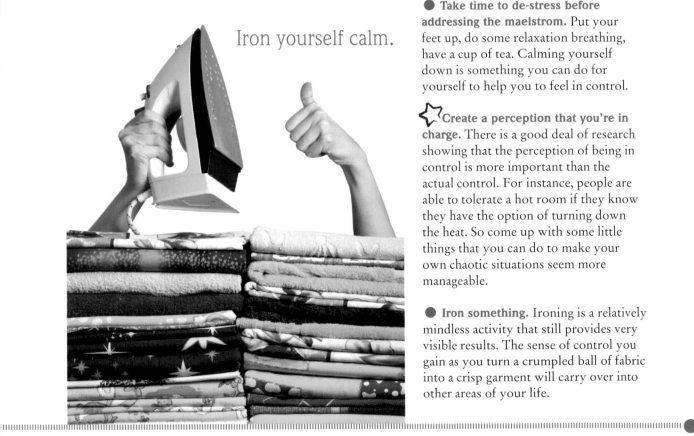

Iron yourself calm.

● **Build up tolerance to chaos** by giving yourself small out-of-control experiences. For instance, if you are typically the main driver of the family car, ask your partner to take the wheel next time you all go out together. Ask someone to interrupt you periodically, invite your partner to make the weekend plans without your input, turn over the bill paying to your partner. These will help you to learn to accept being out of control.

▶ **Practise positive self-talk.** It would be great if someone else did this for you, but often you have to do it for yourself. Self-talk means saying things like, 'I'm going to be OK', 'I'll get through this' or 'Right now, I have to give myself a few minutes, then I can begin coming up with a plan to handle this.'

● **Take time to de-stress before addressing the maelstrom.** Put your feet up, do some relaxation breathing, have a cup of tea. Calming yourself down is something you can do for yourself to help you to feel in control.

☆**Create a perception that you're in charge.** There is a good deal of research showing that the perception of being in control is more important than the actual control. For instance, people are able to tolerate a hot room if they know they have the option of turning down the heat. So come up with some little things that you can do to make your own chaotic situations seem more manageable.

● **Iron something.** Ironing is a relatively mindless activity that still provides very visible results. The sense of control you gain as you turn a crumpled ball of fabric into a crisp garment will carry over into other areas of your life.

Enhancing your sense of **HUMOUR**

What is the greatest reward of being alive? Is it chocolate, sex, ice cream, exotic holidays, hugs, a perfect night's sleep or the satisfaction of a job well done? A thousand people, a thousand different answers. But one supreme pleasure that everyone shares is laughter. Little can compare to the feeling of a deep, complete, heartfelt bout of laughter. No matter your age, wealth, race or lifestyle, things are good when laughter is frequent. Life is also healthier. Research finds that humour can help you to cope better with pain, enhance your immune system, reduce stress and even help you to live longer. Here are our 17 health-boosting tips for getting – or developing – your sense of humour.

17 WAYS TO BRING OUT THE LAUGHTER INSIDE YOU

Improving your
MEMORY

Five things you need to buy at the supermarket – forgotten. The name of your neighbour's son – lost. The magazine you wanted to show a colleague – left at home. Relax. These little memory meltdowns are an inevitable part of life. In most cases, they have nothing to do with Alzheimer's, nothing to do with disease or injury, and everything to do with stress, too much work and daily chaos. The good news is that there has been massive research into the origins and maintenance of memory. If you think you have a serious memory decline, seek medical attention, of course. But if you're just trying to have fewer 'senior moments', you'll find some help in the following 25 tips.

25 TRICKS TO KEEP YOUR BRAIN IN SHAPE

Use it or lose it: the golden rule of brainpower. The brain functions like a muscle in that the more you use it, the stronger it gets. Watching lots of unstimulating TV, having a routine job, cooking, cleaning and shopping the same way over and over – all contribute to a loss of brainpower. Learning new things, varying your routines, having provocative discussions, going on exciting trips and playing a musical instrument all cause your brain to make new connections and function better.

Take a B-complex vitamin pill. As you age, your body becomes less efficient at absorbing certain B vitamins from food. Yet the Bs are critical for maintaining a sharp memory. A study of 260 healthy men and women over the age of 60 found that those with low blood levels of vitamins C or B_{12} scored the worst on memory and cognitive functioning tests. Those with low levels of the B vitamins riboflavin or folic acid scored worst on a test of abstract thinking. Another study found that giving women a B-complex supplement improved their performance on memory tests. B vitamins also help to lower levels of artery-clogging homocysteine, linked to memory loss. Two other supplements to take along with your Bs are vitamins E and C. Studies find that taking the two together can protect against Alzheimer's. But taking the supplements separately (for example, one in the morning and one at night) had no effect.

Put whole-grain bread back into your diet. If you've been following a high-protein, low-carb diet and simultaneously finding your memory going, it's probably not a coincidence. More than any other organ, the brain relies on glucose for fuel. And glucose comes from carbs.

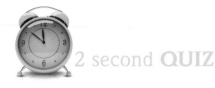
One study of 22 older people from the University of Toronto found that those whose diets contained the greatest percentage of calories as carbohydrates performed best on memory and task tests. Make sure you're getting your carbs from fruits, vegetables and whole grains, not ice cream, sweets and cake.

Take up oil painting. Or fishing, or needlework, or ballroom dancing, or piano. The idea here is to continue stretching your mind around new things and new experiences, which studies find can help to stave off dementia and improve memory.

Eat oil-rich fish at least once a week. Fresh tuna, salmon, trout and mackerel are high in omega-3 fatty acids, important for maintaining memory. A delicious fresh tuna salad, for example, is a real brain treat. (However, canned tuna contains little or no omega-3s).

Eat a vegetarian dinner at least once a week. Low in saturated fat and high in fibre, a veggie meal will boost your efforts to maintain healthy cholesterol levels. That's important in terms of the memory, because high cholesterol levels eventually damage blood vessels, affecting long-term memory and speeding the progression of Parkinson's and Alzheimer's diseases.

Learn new skills like oil painting.

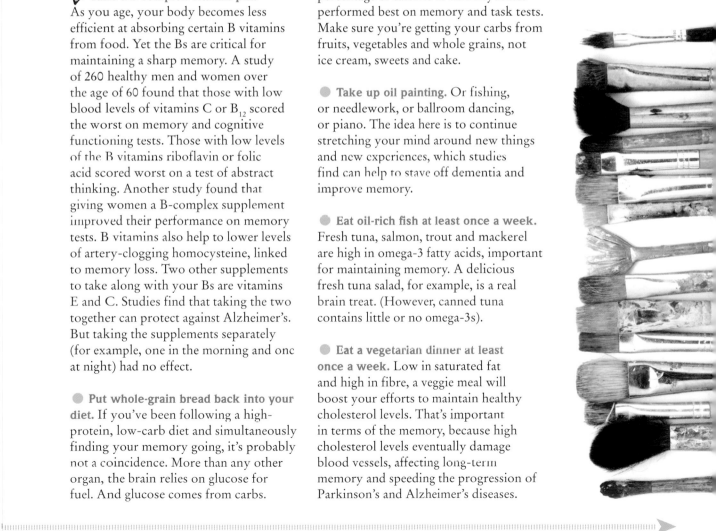

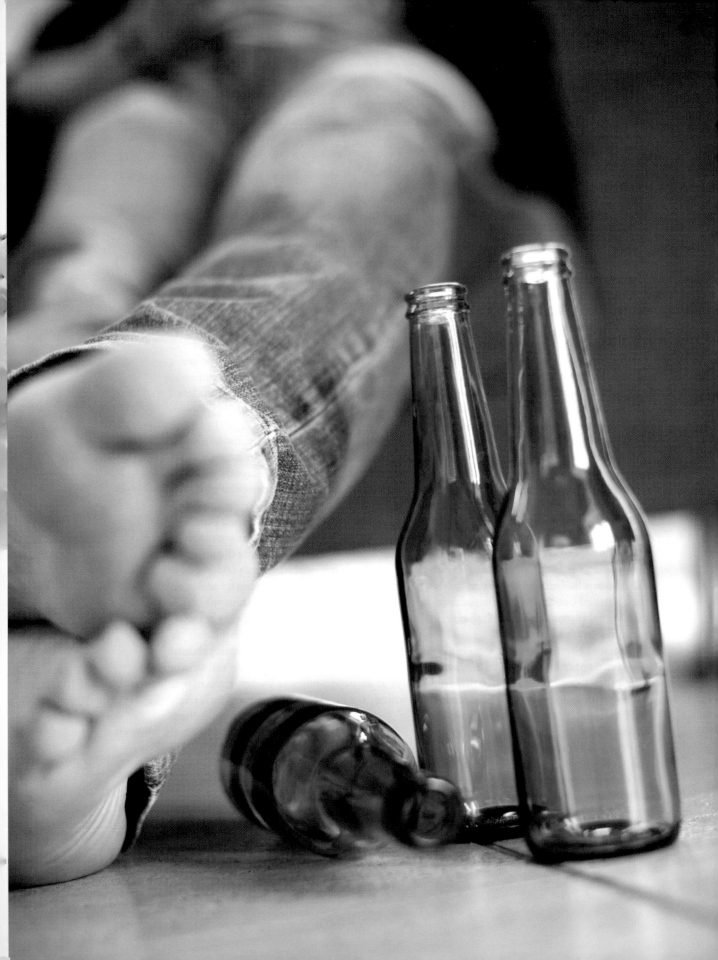

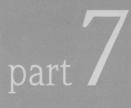

part 7

HABIT CONTROL

It's not the occasional binge or bender that causes lasting damage – it's the unhealthy habits we indulge in every day. Here's some practical advice for kicking bad habits that affect your long-term health.

Give any extra TVs to charity. Allow your home one TV in a room dedicated to nothing but reading or TV watching. Donate the rest to a school or charitable organisation in your community. You'll feel good, but it will be that much harder to veg out in front of the TV.

Turn on the TV only to watch a particular programme. In other words, don't just turn it on and go surfing for something worthwhile. Hours are quickly wasted, jumping from one show to the next, watching all and none at the same time. And, if your TV works without the remote, rather than surf, get up to change channels on the set.

Then, when you sit down to watch a particular programme, set a timer or an alarm clock in another room for the length of the show. When it beeps, you'll have to get out of your chair to turn it off, a signal to turn off the TV as well.

Set a rule that you can't watch TV or surf the internet if the sun is shining. Instead, you have to go for a walk, ride a bike or get some other kind of healthy physical activity for at least an hour before you can turn on the TV or PC. This rule also works well for your children or grandchildren.

Rearrange the furniture. Design your family room so that the television is no longer the focal point of the room, but an afterthought that requires twisting round or rearranging chairs to view it.

Hide the television. Put it behind a screen, hang a cover over it or stick it inside a cabinet. Do whatever you can to ensure it fades into the background and can't be seen when it's off.

Eat meals, especially dinner, with the television and computer firmly OFF. And ensure that every family member knows that eating at the computer is a no-no at any time. That goes for games consoles as well.

Make a TV-watching plan each week. Sit down with the viewing guide and pick out the programmes you want to watch that week. View only those programmes and, when they're over, turn the TV off.

Set surfing, MSN and Facebook limits. Social networks have transformed computer use among the young, and adults are now fast catching on. Or you may just love to blog, check news websites or search for books or holidays. Time flies. But set yourself limits – no more than an hour an evening, say. And then try to do something more physical.

Make a rule that you must read 30 pages of a book or magazine before you can turn on the TV or PC. Pick the right reading matter and you'll soon find you've created a new addiction.

Create a list of 1 hour evening projects. List everything you can possibly dream of: cleaning a particularly messy cupboard, organising recipes, touching up the paint on your bedroom walls,

Healthy **INVESTMENT**

Knitting needles and a ball of wool
Learn to knit while you watch television; it will keep you from eating your way through the evening, and you'll accomplish something productive.

sharpening kitchen knives, sorting through your sewing materials. Then try to do one each evening.

🖵 **Choose games.** With your partner and/or children, relearn the fun of Scrabble, backgammon or chess. Get out the playing cards and have a snap or gin rummy battle. Play table tennis, pool or darts. Go outside and work on your golf swing with practice balls. All of these are more fun, healthy and life-affirming than sitting in front of a TV or computer.

▕▕▐▶ Develop a fast-moving news routine. Most news programmes are scheduled down to the minute. So investigate the handful of programmes you watch and figure out when they run the features you are most interested in, for example, the local weather, the recap of the day's headlines or the sports news. Watch when you get home, then turn off the television for the rest of the night.

🖵 **Say no to watching *Jaws* – yet again.** Often we can be strangely drawn into watching things we've seen many times before. There's something comforting in the repetition. Well, resist it. Viewing the same thing again and again is unhealthy for your body and your brain.

🖵 **Get outdoors every night.** Make a point of leaving your home at least once after dinner, if only for a short walk. Too many of us consider the day pretty much done once we've eaten dinner when, in fact, evening can be a wonderful time for having fun, particularly on long summer evenings.

🖵 **Change your TV-viewing chairs.** Make them somewhat hard and upright – chairs you don't want to lounge in for hours. Move your most comfy chairs to the living room, for listening to music and reading.

> Make the most of those long summer evenings.

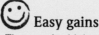

Reminder

▕▕▐▶ Fast results
These are tips that deliver benefits particularly quickly – in some cases, immediately.

☺ Easy gains
These are health boosters that offer the best value for the least amount of effort.

☆ Super-effective
This is advice that scientific research or widespread usage by experts has shown to be especially effective.

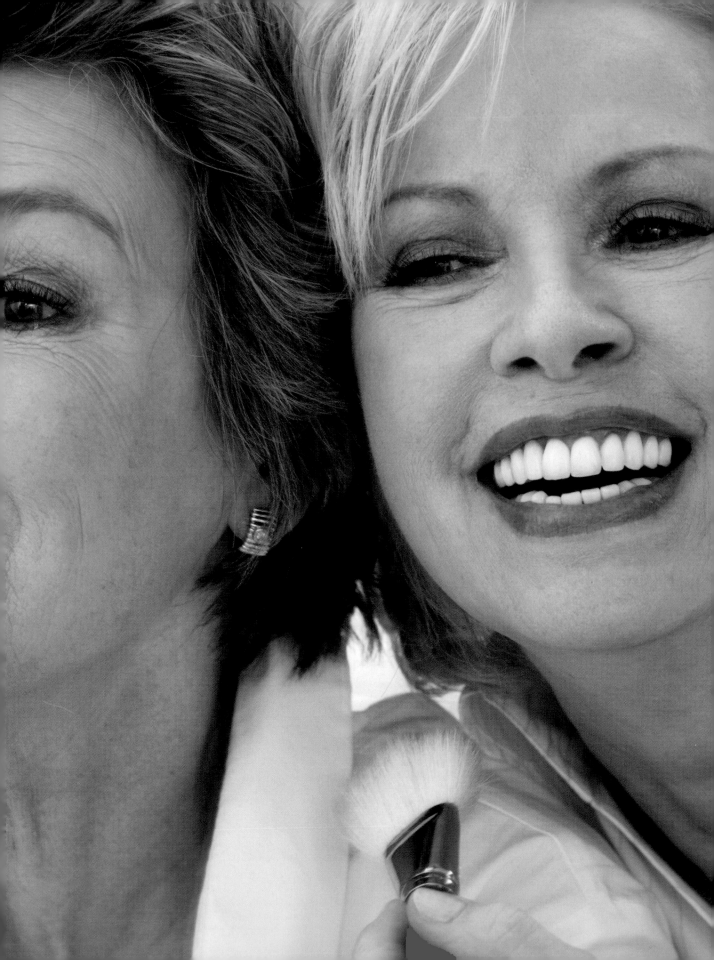

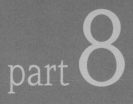
part 8

HEALTH BOOSTING LOOKS

Let's be honest. Looking good feels good. But appearance isn't just about vanity; healthy skin and teeth contribute to overall health. Here are easy, fast ways to look your best.

Healthy SKIN

Beauty, the saying goes, is only skin-deep. But the importance of skin goes a lot deeper. In particular, your skin is the first layer of your immune system, serving as a shield between you and legions of germs. And, of course, your sense of touch is crucial for everyday functions. Like any part of your internal body, though, your skin can be healthy or ill. In particular, ageing causes the skin to become thinner and drier. While you can't control your age, you can control numerous other factors, such as a poor diet and cigarette smoking. Unlike your other organs, you can apply medicines, moisturisers and other potions directly to your skin. So, there's absolutely no reason why you can't have good skin throughout your life, especially if you follow these 37 health-boosting tips.

37 QUICK TRICKS TO ENHANCE YOUR GLOW

● **Skip long, steamy showers** and opt for shorter, cooler sprays. Long, hot showers strip skin of its moisture and wash away the protective oils. So limit your showers to 10 minutes and keep the water cool.

▶ **Check the dryness of your skin** by scratching a small area on your arm or leg with your fingernail. If it leaves a white mark, your skin is indeed dry and needs both moisture and exfoliation (that is, removal of the outermost layer of dead skin cells).

● **Treat your neck and chest like an extension of your face.** Your neck and upper chest area is covered by very sensitive skin, making it a prime spot for telltale signs of ageing such as dryness. To keep this area youthful, use facial cleansing creams that hydrate and cleanse gently rather than deodorant soaps, which can be drying. Top it all off with a good facial moisturising cream. If this area is extra dry, use a facial moisturising mask twice a month.

☺ **Run a humidifier every night in winter** to moisturise the air in your bedroom. Not only will it ease itchy, dry skin, but you'll be able to breathe the moist air more easily.

▶ **Switch from a deodorant soap to a special moisturising product,** such as Dove, Oilatum or Neutrogena. Deodorant soaps can be drying, whereas these specially designed products leave an oily, yet beneficial, film on your skin.

● **Keep your beauty products simple,** particularly if you have sensitive skin. Stay away from anything with colour or fragrance, or anything that produces bubbles or has 'antibacterial' on the label.

Do **THREE** things...

If you do only three things to improve the look and feel of your skin, make them these three, agree several of our experts:

1 Drink at least eight 250ml glasses of water a day to stay hydrated. This helps to flush toxins through your kidneys instead of your skin.

2 Follow a healthy diet rich in fruits, vegetables and fish. When researchers from Monash University in Australia studied the diets of 453 people aged 70 and older from Australia, Greece and Sweden to see if there was any correlation between what they ate and the number of wrinkles in their skin, they found that those who ate the most fruit, vegetables and fish had the fewest wrinkles. Conversely, the researchers found, foods high in saturated fat, including meat, butter and full-fat dairy products, as well as soft drinks, cakes, pastries and potatoes, increased the likelihood of skin wrinkling.

3 Protect your skin from the sun all year round with a sunblock that has an SPF of 30 or greater. Just because there's snow on the ground doesn't mean your skin can't be damaged by the sun. Time outdoors is time well spent, but be sure to keep your skin either well covered or well protected with sunblock. In particular, the sun is at its most damaging between 11am and 3pm.

● **Smooth a couple of drops of olive oil over your face, elbows, knees and the backs of your arms** every evening. The oil contains monounsaturated fat, which refreshes and hydrates the skin without leaving a greasy residue.

● **For soft, young-looking hands and feet,** put on plenty of moisturising cream, then slip on thin fabric socks and gloves while you sleep.

● **Tone your skin with a sage,** peppermint and witch hazel combination. Sage helps to control oil, peppermint creates a cool tingle, and witch hazel helps to restore the skin's protective layer.

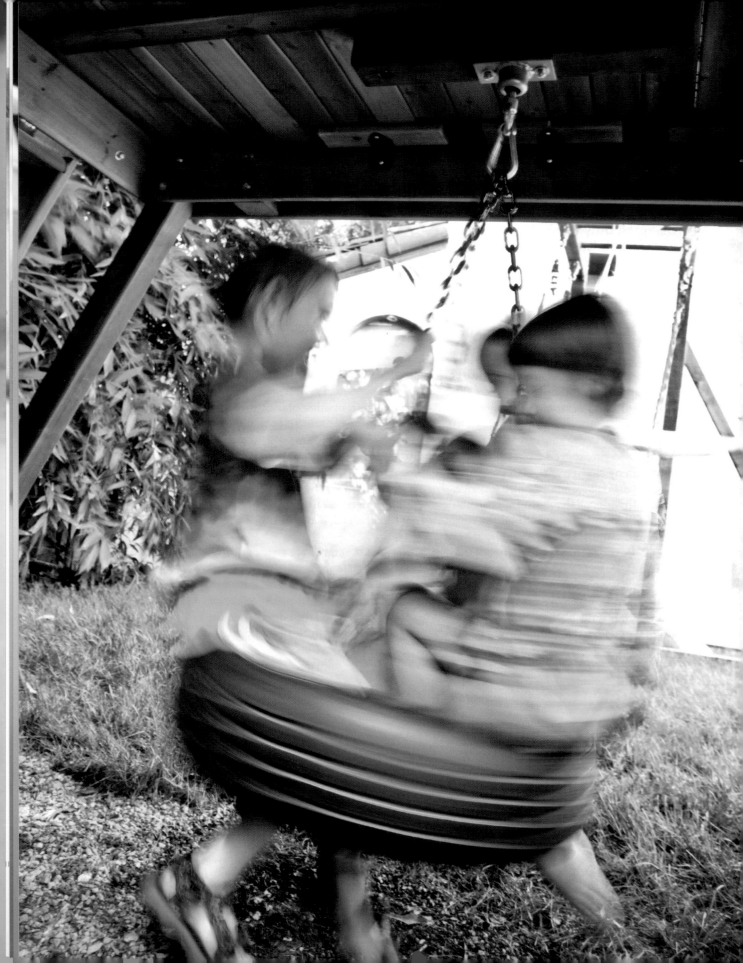

part 9

PEOPLE & PLACES

Your relationships have a very real effect on your physical health. Here's how to make sure the people around you are helping – not hurting – your well-being.

discuss difficult parenting issues. Your bed is a place for good things only – sleep, companionship, romance. If it becomes a place for hard talks and criticism, one of you will eventually feel your bedroom is emotionally unsafe, and you'll start to avoid each other. If this is already going on, you need to stop it – declare the bedroom a safe zone, and make sure all serious discussions take place earlier and elsewhere.

● **Pursue your own interests.** Go ahead, take that writing class – or pursue any other interest you might have outside those you share with your partner. It makes you more interesting to your partner and everyone else. Moreover, a little 'me time' allows both of you to grow as individuals and reduces the pressure on each of you to fill the other's every need.

● **Take a weekend getaway.** If you present the idea to your partner as an adventure, he or she'll be more inclined to get in on the act. Then the fun begins: deciding where you'll go, what you'll do, and how you'll get there. Plan it together. Pore over maps and the travel section of the newspaper together. Discuss whether you should splash out on a room with a hot tub or a four-poster.

● **Renew your vows.** Renewing your vows renews your commitment not only to your partner but also to keeping passion and intimacy in your relationship. You can do it once a year by taking a romantic getaway on your anniversary or make it a once-in-a-lifetime event.

● **Read the cartoons out loud to each other** and share funny stories. A 2004 study found that sharing humorous experiences significantly reduced the amount of conflict couples felt.

● **Go shopping (or watch a football match) with a close friend.** One study found that couples who have individual friendships outside their relationship were more satisfied with their marital relationships than those who didn't.

● **Demonstrate your love by trying to improve something about yourself** that upsets your partner. For instance, if your partner likes order and tidiness, stop throwing your dirty socks on the floor and leaving your dishes in the sink. Saying 'I love you' is always nice, but showing it is really fundamental.

☆ **Always put your marriage first,** even if you have a houseful of children. This is a golden rule: of all your relationships, your partner must come first. After all, the children are going to leave some day; hopefully, your partner isn't. Plus, giving up your life as a couple to indulge your children simply sets an uninspiring example: grow up, become an adult, then you, too, can subjugate your existence to that of your children. Putting your marriage first means things like deliberately setting aside time for the two of you, whether it's a weekly date, a nightly bath together or dinner alone a few nights a week (feed the children early).

Healthy INVESTMENT

A CD you both love
One study found that when couples listened to music they both liked, they felt more caring towards their partner. It's just something else they can share.

Your **CHILDREN**

You remember them in nappies. You recall their first words. You cherish the days when they were innocent, loving and eager for your hugs. And yet, as your children grow and evolve, so must your relationship with them. You need to be supportive but not intrusive; offer emotional back-up without being overly involved in their lives; and hope they make wise choices, while understanding that those choices are theirs to make. The tips that follow can help you to bond with your children even if they're no longer children. This, too, is a matter of health: nothing can break your heart as much as a strained relationship with your child. And nothing can make your heart soar as much as watching their lives prosper – and them wanting you to be part of it.

13 WAYS TO SUSTAIN THE LOVE AND RESPECT

8 great ways
TO GET CLOSER

1 Teach older parents to use email or surf the internet.

2 Introduce your parents to your friends, and include them in social gatherings when appropriate.

3 Eat out together. Try a cuisine you've never tried before.

4 Join a book or investment club together.

5 Read the same books and talk about them in your own book club.

6 Start a new family tradition with the grandchildren, such as once-a-month picnics.

7 Challenge your parents to a round of golf or a hand of gin rummy.

8 Go bike riding or for a walk together.

● **Create opportunities for exploring and uncovering memories.** If your parents are older, look through their photo albums with them, asking them for stories about the people in the photos. You can help your parents to discover the meaning in their lives by encouraging them to talk about their accomplishments, the high points, and their joys and sorrows.

● **Help your parents to preserve their memories on film, CD or in a scrapbook.** The finished product will not only be a testament to a renewed closeness between you, but also provides a wonderful legacy.

● **Express your appreciation for all your parents have done for you.** Yes, they may do things that annoy you, but they also come to your rescue when you need help.

The point is, your parents still do things for you that deserve your notice – and your gratitude.

● **Rediscover and share mutual interests.** When you were a child, did you and your dad share a passion for a particular football team? Did you and your mum spend time each summer making jam? Make these happy memories the foundation for new, shared activities.

● **Be honest about who you are and what you want.** Maybe there are things about the way you grew up that your parents regret. But as long as *you* don't regret anything, they have to adjust. Be clear about who you want to be and help your parents to accept you as you are.

● **Do not allow them to channel guilt at you.** If your parents are the type to complain about you never calling, never visiting, forgetting an uncle's birthday, not sending enough pictures or whatever irks them that day, don't take the bait and feel guilty – unless you honestly regret the oversight. In which case, apologise immediately and seek a way to make amends. Otherwise, let it wash over you. You are a mature, independent adult, and you act on your own volition. For more on this, see 'Dealing with guilt', page 290.

● **Grant them their independence too.** Sometimes it's the grown-up child who doesn't want to cut off the nurturing relationship. If you are past 25 and still find it necessary to talk to your mum every night, or immediately turn to your dad for a house repair rather than your partner, or automatically assume your parents will babysit the children whenever you need to go out, then you may be the problem, not your parents. They deserve freedom too.

NEIGHBOURS and FRIENDS

Modern life is a lot less conducive to friendships and neighbourliness than it used to be. The average person in the UK moves house three or four times. And, these days, we often drive everywhere instead of walking and spend time in front of the TV or computer instead of socialising. Often, we don't even know our neighbours' names. We don't usually realise how much we depend on good neighbours and friends until we lose them. They make our lives more pleasant and give us a sense of who we are. And all it takes to enhance your relationship with them is respect for their feelings, concern for their property and a willingness to offer a helping hand when it's needed. Here's how to nurture your relationships with two types of vitally important people in your life.

10 WAYS TO MAINTAIN A HEALTHY CIRCLE AROUND YOU

COLLEAGUES

You can pick your friends, but you can't pick your colleagues. Yet you need them in more ways than one. First, you need their goodwill and cooperation in order to perform your own job well. Second, studies find that disagreements with colleagues and bad working relationships deflate morale and impair performance even more than rumours of redundancies. And third, if you're like most people, you spend more waking hours at work than anywhere else. Reaching out to your colleagues – or extending an olive branch, if need be – can make your work environment a much nicer place in which to spend so many hours a day. You don't have to be friends with your colleagues, but you do need to be friendly. Read on for fresh ways to make work a happier place to be.

16 WAYS TO KEEP THE PEACE AND HAVE FUN AT WORK

☺ **Say a cheery 'Hello!' in the morning.** Do you plod into the office, eyes down, shoulders slumped, and immediately start work? If so, you're likely to find that colleagues ignore you (at best) or avoid you (at worst). Get into the habit of smiling and greeting everyone as you arrive in the morning or begin your shift. It's amazing how fast this little courtesy can thaw chilly workplace relations.

● **Learn the art of small talk.** Ask your colleagues about their interests – their favourite music, films, books, hobbies. Showing a genuine interest in them will make them feel comfortable around you.

● **Join the office sports team.** Many offices have a sports team, be it football, cricket, tennis or rounders, and joining in is a great way to enjoy some exercise while you get to know your colleagues in an informal setting.

● **Accept good-natured teasing.** Other workers sometimes play jokes and tease to test what kind of person you are. So if they poke fun at your new shoes or mischievously put a funny screensaver on your computer, don't get angry. Let them know that you enjoy a good joke – even if it's sometimes on you. Of course, if the teasing is personal (about your weight or ethnicity, for example), and makes it difficult for you to do your job or makes you feel uncomfortable because of its sexual implications, you may need to take up the matter with your supervisor.

● **Ask what they think.** People love to be asked their opinion, so go out of your way to ask, 'What do you think is missing from this report?' or 'How do you think I should handle this situation with X?' Then give the advice-giver a sincere thank you, even if the ideas are less than helpful.

In PERSPECTIVE

Office friendships benefit your work

Do you have a best pal at work? Chances are, if you do, you're a better, more productive worker than the office loner or grouch, research shows.

If you have a strong office friendship, you're more likely to be engaged with your work. And a 2009 UK Gallup poll finds that a sense of engagement really matters. According to Gallup, 60 per cent of employees without a good pal are not engaged, and 36 per cent are actively disengaged. Only 4 per cent of those without a good work friend are content and productive at work. Engaged employees are those who know what's expected of them and who have what they need in order to do their job. They also feel that they are involved in making a difference, along with colleagues whom they can trust. Not only that, they have chances to improve and develop at work.

At the opposite end of the spectrum are people described as CAVE dwellers – Consistently Against Virtually Everything – the people who are actively disengaged at work. Unfortunately, these negative people are often the most vocal.

The advice to employers to ensure their employees feel engaged is to work at raising and maintaining morale, hope and trust among workers, to concentrate on employees' strengths and to improve workplace communication.

☆ **Avoid gossip.** You don't want anyone talking about you behind your back, so return the favour. When a colleague sidles up to you bearing a juicy titbit of gossip about an office romance or someone's impending dismissal, respond with, 'Really?', then change the subject or get back to work. If you don't respond, the gossiper will move on – and you'll retain the trust and respect of your colleagues.

▐▶ **When dealing with a difficult colleague,** pretend your children are watching. This simple visualisation technique will help you to keep a cool head. After all, you've taught your children to have good manners. With them 'watching', it will be difficult to stoop to the level of your infuriating colleague.

2 second QUIZ

Show your emotions or keep your cool?
ANSWER: **KEEP YOUR COOL.**

A US study in 2002 found that many employees don't want their colleagues to express any type of strong emotion – positive or negative – on the job.

● **Ladle out the compliments.** Did Tom fix the office photocopier – again? Has Ann stopped smoking? By all means, compliment your colleagues on their achievements – personal or professional. Too often, we focus on what people are doing wrong.

● **Spread your good cheer.** You don't have to be a Pollyanna, but try to perform one kindly act a week, choosing a different colleague each time. For example, one week you might bring in cakes for no reason. Another week, it might be a card for a colleague – maybe a thank-you note for helping you out the week before, or a light, humorous card for a colleague who seems to be a bit down.

● **Return calls and emails promptly.** To win friends at work, a good place to start is good office etiquette. There's nothing more frustrating to busy people than to have their emails and phone messages ignored. Your silence doesn't just make their job harder to do; it also conveys an unpleasant message to them: you're unimportant to me.

● **Give credit where credit is due.** Don't withhold credit from deserving colleagues. You'll alienate them, and they won't be there for you when you need them (or when they all go out for lunch). Embrace the attitude that we all win together, and let others know when someone has done something above and beyond the call of duty on a project. Also, if someone incorrectly gives you credit and praise, acknowledge your colleague who does deserve the accolades. It will be remembered.

● **Here's one for the boss:** always work at least as hard as anyone working with or for you. Make it clear that you would never ask anyone to do a level of work you wouldn't be willing to take on yourself.

● **Always be on time** to show you respect other people's time.

● **Express your good ideas** in a way that makes it clear that they are not the only good ideas, and that others may have equally good insights to add.

● **Talk about your life outside the office when it's appropriate.** This will remind the people you work with that you're a person first, not just an employee or employer.

Assume the positive about what you don't know. Isn't it funny how a team of workers often think they're working harder than another team elsewhere in the building? Or that the bosses are clueless? Don't subscribe to that kind of toxic thinking, even if it's rampant. It's a negative attitude that makes work become miserable. Instead, assume that everyone else is working hard and doing their best, even if you don't know what their work is. You should believe both in the work you're doing and the organisation you're doing it for. If you can't, perhaps it's time to move on.

On an
AEROPLANE

There's only one way really to enjoy flying: buy your own plane.
The rest of us are stuck with missed and cancelled flights, tightly packed cabins and humiliating security procedures, all of which are enough to send stress levels soaring. Add to that the physical tolls extracted by cabin air that's literally drier than the air in the Sahara, the changing cabin pressure and the hours of sitting in a chair barely wider than your hips, with someone's seat back in your lap, and you'll understand why the following health-boosting tips are so critical when you take to the skies.

16 STRATEGIES FOR A HEALTHY FLIGHT

☺ **Pack three camomile tea bags in your hand luggage.** When the flight attendant comes round with drinks, ask for a cup of hot water and dunk in your tea bag. The herbal tea will soothe any travel jitters and relax you enough to get some sleep on the plane, ensuring you arrive refreshed.

✈ **Use a carry-on backpack so that you can take the stairs** in the airport instead of the lift or escalator. You'll probably have the stairs all to yourself, and it's a great way to stretch your legs and burn a few calories before you get on-board. As you wait for your flight, power walk through the terminal. You can rack up a couple of miles just by striding to and from the gates and circling the baggage carousel.

✈ **Buy a pair of flight socks.** You can purchase special flight socks (called compression stockings), which improve blood flow during the journey, helping to relieve aching legs and prevent deep vein thrombosis (DVT). Make sure you choose the correct size, not just for your foot, but for your ankle and calf. The socks should not be too loose or restrictive or cause you any discomfort or pain.

✈ **Get up and walk between meals, and use that time to stretch.** Do the following stretching exercises at least once every hour during the flight:
● Standing in the aisle, stretch your calves by taking a large step back with one leg and reaching into the floor with your back heel.
● Also while standing, stretch your torso and back by twisting gently from side to side.
● Then, when seated, stretch your arms, shoulders and upper back by extending one arm overhead, bending it and placing your palm against your shoulder blade. You can use the other arm to increase the stretch.

▐▶ **In your seat, perform these six exercises every half-hour.** They will keep the blood flowing and help to prevent stiffness.
● Raise your shoulders and rotate them front to back, then back to front.
● Drop your chin to your chest. Nod yes, then shake no, pointing your chin to one shoulder, then the other.
● Clasp your fingers together, palms facing each other, then stretch your arms out straight in front of you, palms facing out.
● With your heels on the floor, pull your toes up as far as possible. Hold for a few seconds, then release.

In PERSPECTIVE

Jet lag

Nothing's worse than arriving at your holiday destination only to spend the first three days feeling like you've been hit by a truck as you try to recover from jet lag. To reset your internal clock more quickly, follow this advice:
● Allow a day for every time zone you've passed through to recover fully from your jet lag.
● If you're flying east, book an early flight. If you're flying west, however, book a later flight.
● Begin preparing for time changes a few days before your departure by getting up half an hour to an hour earlier or by going to bed later (depending on where you're heading).
● When you get on the plane, immediately adjust your watch to the time of your destination. If it's night-time, try to sleep.
● Use sunlight to reset your clock. After flying west, spend a few hours outdoors in the afternoon; after heading east, take a half-hour walk outside in the morning.

- Lift one foot slightly off the floor and make small circular motions in each direction with your foot. Repeat with the other foot.
- Lift one heel as high as possible while keeping your toes on the floor. Hold for a few seconds, then release. Repeat with the other foot.

✈ **Avoid sitting with your legs crossed.** Instead, prop up your feet on a carry-on bag to make yourself more comfortable.

✈ **If you can, travel business class.** The usual fabric seats in economy class are havens for dust mites and other allergens and germs. The seats in business class are often leather, which is more hygienic.

▐▌▌▶ **Bring a fully charged mobile phone** pre-programmed with airline reservation telephone numbers. If your flight is delayed or cancelled, you can immediately call reservations to rebook. This is much quicker (and less stressful) than standing in the customer-service queue.

✈ **Carry a large, empty plastic coffee cups** (the kind with a top you can sip through). On the plane, ask the attendant to fill it with water. Much better than the tiny cups they usually provide.

✈ **When booking flights, book the first flight of the day.** Particularly if you're flying east (see advice on jet lag, opposite) It's most likely to be on time, so you're less likely to get stressed. An early flight is also more likely to be freshly cleaned.

✈ **Keep your nasal passages and ears clear** by taking a decongestant as directed for 24 hours before your flight. This will shrink the membranes in your sinuses and ears, reducing the painful pressured sensation flying can often produce.

✈ **Chew some chewing gum,** swallow vigorously or yawn widely when the plane is taking off or landing. This will equalise the pressure in your middle ear.

✈ **Skip the alcohol during the flight.** The air in the plane is dry enough; alcohol just dehydrates you even more. It's the same for caffeinated drinks. Water is best.

✈ **Bring a bag of healthy snacks** in your hand luggage even for what should in theory be a short flight. And buy a bottle of water once you're through security. Not only do fewer airlines serve complimentary food these days, but unexpected delays (such as sitting on the tarmac for 90 minutes while the wings of the plane are being de-iced) can send your blood sugar plummeting.

✈ **Resist the temptation to remove your shoes during the flight.** You'll end up with swollen feet due to the low air pressure in the cabin, and your shoes will be uncomfortable when you have to put them back on.

✈ **Dress in layers.** Planes are often too hot or too cold. Stay in control of your own temperature by wearing layers that you can put on or take off.

The bigger the cup, the more water you'll drink.

In a **HOTEL**

Let's say you're lucky enough to take two weeks' holiday away from home each year. Or perhaps your job sends you on a training course for a few days. Then there's your niece's wedding, a weekend getaway or two to the country – or Paris or further afield. All in all, we may spend 10 to 20 nights a year in a hotel room. That's not to be sneezed at. Or, more accurately, that's a lot to sneeze at. We'd all love to stay at five-star hotels with top security and immaculate cleanliness, but the reality is most of us can afford only smaller, cheaper hotels – and hygiene and cleanliness may not be quite up to par. Here are 16 ideas on how to make your holiday home more pleasant, healthier and safer.

16 WAYS TO STAY HEALTHIER AND SAFER

Choose modern over old. Yes, Victorian bed and breakfasts are far superior in terms of charm and personal touches, but their rooms and public sitting areas also tend to accumulate more allergens and dust. So if health is a real concern while travelling, go for good modern hotels.

● **Pack a long-sleeved pyjama top and long PJ trousers.** If you are concerned about the hygiene of bedding in a budget hotel, reduce contact by wearing body-covering PJs and light socks to bed.

Use your bed for sleeping only. Don't work or eat on it and don't watch TV on it. Not only is this more hygienic, but you'll probably find it easier to fall asleep.

● **Ask for an allergy-free room.** Some hotels offer rooms that are designed to minimise the amounts of dust mites and other allergens. Even if you don't have allergies, this might be a good choice if you're prone to colds and flus. Other hotels provide allergy packs, including face masks, special pillows and mattress covers. But you have to ask for them.

● **Ask for a room on the third floor or higher.** Most thefts occur on the first two floors.

● **Divide your breakfast and lunch breaks in two.** Whether away on holiday or business, use half the time for eating and the other half for walking outside. Just as you should always do.

● **If you're staying for several days, book a hotel with a pool or gym room.** Exercising will ease any stiffness from travelling and burn off some of the calories from the breakfast buffet, business lunch or wedding cake.

2 second QUIZ

A hotel or a busy relative's home?
ANSWER: **HOTEL.**

But it's about relationships rather than cleanliness. If you plan to stay for a single night or two, a busy relative will no doubt be delighted to see you but for longer stays it is often better to find a nearby hotel or Bed & Breakfast and drop in on your relative for meals or go out together for pure enjoyment.

● **Pack insect and pest repellent.** In tropical and sub-tropical countries your hotel room could be invaded by mosquitoes, particularly if it is close to open water. Always take an effective insect repellent (and make sure you've taken any necessary precautions in advance, such as anti-malaria pills). Some people also find that taking 100mg vitamin B_1 or 300mg of brewer's yeast keep mosquitoes at bay – take it in advance as the benefits are only apparent after about a week. In some cheaper hotels you may also need protection against bedbugs which leave itchy welts on the skin. The evidence is tiny bloodstains on pillows or mattress liners and seams. If you see any, you should immediately contact the management, ask for a change of room and make sure it's bedbug clear.

Cover up with a long-sleeved pyjama top and long PJ bottoms.

Sagging mattress or sleeping on the floor?
ANSWER: **THE FLOOR.**

If you have back problems of any kind and the hotel bed has seen better days, pull the mattress onto the floor. You'll get better support and be less likely to wake up with a crick in your back that could cramp your style for days.

Keep bugs at bay with a pair of flip-flops.

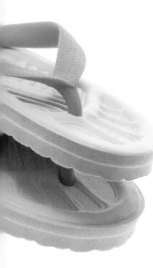

● **Check your luggage for alien bugs and insects when you get home.** If you find any, put your clothes straight into the washing machine, then dry them on high heat for at least 15 minutes. Anything that isn't washable should be put into the freezer for a couple of days.

☺ **Moisten the dry air with the help of a kettle.** If your room has a kettle, fill it with plenty of water, heat it until it steams, then let the steam escape into the room until the water's almost gone. Your sinuses will thank you.

● **Pack a photograph of someone you love (even your dog).** If, when you come back to your room after a stressful day, you begin to feel lonely or get that 'What city am I in?' confusion that often comes with long trips, you can cheer yourself up by looking at the picture and reminding yourself of home.

● **Use your mobile or a battery-operated travel alarm.** You'll fall asleep quicker and sleep better if you don't have to worry about missing an important appointment because you set the hotel alarm wrongly or someone on reception has forgotten your wake-up call.

● **Pack a pair of flip-flops.** Use them in the bathroom, on the carpet (who knows the last time the carpet was properly cleaned) and in the pool area to prevent any fungal (or worse) infections.

● **Be wary of a hotel's hot tub.** There's no doubt that hot tubs are luxuriously soothing and, if you're fit and healthy, go ahead and plunge in. Just be aware that hot tubs can foster bacteria such as the one that causes folliculitis (itchy red bumps). And occasionally people have developed bronchitis and even serious forms of pneumonia from breathing in air contaminated by bacteria in the water.

● **Play it safe.** One of the easiest ways to stay healthy is to make sure that you're not physically attacked in a strange place. Here are some important tips on how to protect yourself when staying in a hotel:
● When registering, make sure the receptionist doesn't say your room number aloud, but instead writes it down and hands it to you. If he or she does say it out loud, ask for another room and ask for the number to be written down.
● If someone knocks on your door, ask who it is and verify before opening. If you didn't order room service, or don't know why the 'employee' is there, call the front desk to verify they sent someone.
● Use the main entrance of the hotel when returning in the evening.
● Use all of the locking devices for your door, and lock all of the windows and sliding glass doors.

● **Don't leave the 'Please Clean the Room' sign** outside your door unless you want to tell the whole world you're not there. Instead, put the 'Do Not Disturb' sign on the door. If you want your room cleaned while you're out, call reception and let them know.

In the **GARDEN**

Quick: what is one of the best ways to reduce your risk of hypertension, osteoporosis and depression? How about digging in the dirt? Studies find that gardening is one of the best physical activities of all when it comes to preventing or improving chronic health conditions. Plus, the stress-relieving benefits of watching something grow, of breathing in the scent of flowers, of picking a sun-kissed tomato from your own garden, are legion.

The key is not to overdo it or do it incorrectly. These 13 health-boosting tips will enable you to remain healthy while gardening.

13 SECRETS FOR HEALTHIER DIGGING

Electric mower or manual?
ANSWER: **FOR MOST GARDENS, MANUAL.**

You'll get a much better workout every time you cut the grass, and the intensity isn't that great if your garden is small to medium-sized. If you have a larger garden, you can go with an electric or petrol mower, but make it a push, not ride-on, mower.

❀ **Stretch for 5 minutes before heading out to the garden.** Focus on your hamstrings, back and arms. For specific moves, see 'Stretching', page 134.

❀ **Dress for gardening.** That means wearing sunscreen with an SPF of 30 or higher and reapplying it every couple of hours. Also put on insect spray, a hat, sunglasses and a light, long-sleeved shirt that covers most of your neck.

❀ **Bend from your knees and take frequent breaks from bending over.** Back strain is a common gardening injury. Other ways to avoid it are to carry a small stool with you to sit or lean on while weeding, and to use knee pads to protect your kneecaps from hard ground.

❀ **Check the pollen count before heading out,** particularly if you suffer from allergies or asthma. Also, forgo gardening on days of high heat and humidity. The heavy air could cause problems if you have respiratory issues.

❀ **Choose gardening tools with padded handles** to protect the joints in your hands and fingers from excess pressure. Tools such as shears or clippers with a spring-action, self-opening feature are particularly helpful if you have a weak grasp.

❀ **Divide large bags** of mulch, dirt or fertiliser into smaller, more manageable loads and use a trolley or wheelbarrow to move materials. When lifting, use the muscles in your legs, not your back.

❀ **Vary your tasks to avoid overstressing any one part of your body.** For instance, don't spend the entire day stooping and weeding. Instead, pick one section of the garden and complete it: weeding, laying the mulch, then raking. Tackle another section the following day.

❀ **Carry a mobile phone** Garden accidents do occasionally occur. It could be a painful strain or worse. Make sure you could quickly summon help if need be, especially if you're on your allotment away from home.

❀ **Plant at least one vegetable in your garden.** You'll be more likely to eat it. Also plant some herbs to use for flavouring food in place of salt.

❀ **Keep all your gardening tools, gloves,** etc. in a backpack that you can carry with you as you move from bed to bed.

❀ **Keep your garden manageable.** If you take on too much too soon, you'll find you ache the next morning (and risk a more serious injury), and you'll quickly become overwhelmed and stop altogether.

❀ **Carry a water bottle with you** if you're spending the day on an allotment. And be sure to sip on it every 30 minutes or so. It's easy to become dehydrated when you're working outdoors.

❀ **Take time after gardening** to sit in a shady spot and admire your accomplishments. Sip a cool drink and enjoy the beauty around you.

In a **CROWD**

You're seated in a venue with a thousand other people. Which do you feel more threatened by: a fire or a stranger sneezing on you?

The chances are, most of us aren't very concerned about either. Which is an acceptable attitude to have – the first is unlikely, the second poses a relatively minor health risk. But they pose risks nonetheless. And with a little more forethought, you can better protect your health and safety in the rare event that something goes wrong at the concert hall or football match. The advice here is not to avoid crowds. Rather, be sure to follow these tips to keep yourself and your loved ones safe and healthy while you're out living life to the fullest.

11 WAYS TO STAY SAFE AND HEALTHY

Keep your hands in your pockets. The formula for getting ill: germs get on hands, hands touch face, germs enter body, you are infected. Where there are crowds, there are germs – millions of them – on every surface. Don't touch them and they won't make you ill.

● **Carry a bottle of hand sanitiser.** Use it after portaloo visits, before eating and any time you feel contaminated by the microbes of the masses.

● **Put a pair of earplugs in your handbag or pocket.** If the event gets too loud, or you get stuck standing next to the speakers, use the earplugs.

● **Look for the emergency-exit signs as you enter a large venue.** It takes only seconds – and those seconds could turn out to be the most worthwhile ever. One study found that more than half of fatalities at concerts occurred when people were trying to get out of the building or concert setting.

● **Arrange a place to meet** your family or friends in case you get separated. Actually, you should choose two places: one inside and one outside.

● **In the rare event of a stampede,** try to move sideways to the crowd until you get to a wall. Then press yourself against it until the crowd dissipates, or you find a better exit. It doesn't happen often, but people do get trampled to death. If you've memorised the emergency exits, you'll have a better chance of getting to one that the rest of the crowd may not have noticed.

● **Pack your own lunch.** Peanut butter or jam sandwiches and apples will keep for the whole day and will help to forestall your children's pleas for junk food from the vendors at the event site. If you can't avoid buying from food stalls, check out the vendor. Does the stall look clean? Are the cook's hands clean? Is the vendor handling the food with gloves? Does he or she handle money, then touch the food? It's hard to tell just by looking at it if food will make you ill, but you should definitely avoid undercooked (pink) meats and meat that is not hot when served. The last thing you need when you're in a place that only has portaloos is food poisoning.

● **Remember to put a wad of tissues in your handbag or pocket.** Now you have emergency toilet paper if you have to use the portaloos.

● **Put water bottles in the freezer the night before.** You'll save money on overpriced bottled water at the event and, as the ice melts, you'll have nice cold water on hand to stay hydrated.

● **Dress in layers.** The crowd is pressing in around you, you feel overly warm … and suddenly the ground comes up to meet you. Don't let it happen. If you've dressed in layers, you can shed one of them if you get too hot. If you're wearing only one layer to start with, you might just get arrested! Of course, layering your clothing works the other way too. If the temperature drops as the match goes into overtime, you'll be prepared.

● **Sit and wait when the curtain comes down.** Let the crowd go first. You'll get out of the car park more easily and avoid ruining your great time out with a bout of blood pressure-raising stress.

Be prepared – save money and avoid germs by packing your own lunch.

Out in the SNOW

What is it about a snowfall that brings out the child in all of us? Perhaps because it's a bit of a novelty. Suddenly we're ready to bundle up and head outside to play. Plus, snow is great for a midwinter workout, what with all the sledging and snow-clearing you can do. Whether you're outside shovelling your path, driving or just making a snowman, follow the tips here to keep safe and warm.

12 WAYS TO KEEP SAFE AND WARM

● **Apply a Vaseline shield.** If it's cold and windy, your face may suffer a case of windburn. A thin coating of Vaseline on exposed skin – particularly your cheeks, nose, chin, ears and neck – will help to prevent it.

● **Don't walk with your hands in your pockets.** It's pretty basic advice, but that way, you can use your arms to regain your balance if you slip.

In PERSPECTIVE

Frostbite

In the UK, it's not a common winter hazard, but in a period of extreme cold or when you go skiing, frostbite could be a very real threat. Quite often, the worst might be permanent numbness but you can end up with gangrene – and lose a toe, finger, ear or even your nose as a result – if you're not careful. So it's important to recognise symptoms:
● A pins-and-needles sensation, then numbness.
● Hard, pale, cold, numb skin. When frostbitten skin has thawed, it becomes red and painful (early frostbite). More severe frostbite results in white and numb skin.

If you or someone you're with has frostbite:
● Get the person to a warmer place. Remove any constricting jewellery and wet clothing and, if possible, wrap the affected areas in sterile dressings (remember to separate affected fingers and toes) then get the person to the nearest A & E department.
● If immediate care is not available, immerse affected areas in warm – never hot – water or repeatedly apply warm cloths to affected ears, nose or cheeks for 20 to 30 minutes. The warming is complete when the skin is soft and sensation returns.
● Move thawed areas as little as possible.
● If the frostbite is extensive, give warm drinks, but never alcohol, to the person in order to replace lost fluids.
● Don't thaw a frostbitten area if it cannot be kept thawed. Refreezing may make tissue damage even worse. Also, don't use direct dry heat (such as a radiator, campfire, heating pad or hairdryer). Direct heat can burn already-damaged tissues.
● Don't rub the area, or disturb blisters on frostbitten skin.

● **Beware: ice.** If it's icy, wear rubber-soled boots with good traction, go slowly, don't carry too many bags and give yourself extra time to get wherever you're going, whether on foot or in a car.

● **Or buy traction devices for your shoes.** It's possible to buy antislip spikes or stretchable traction devices that fit over your shoes to prevent you from slipping on ice or snow. Yaktrax, for example, are rubber and wire devices that fit over the bottom of your boots. Go to www.yaktrax.co.uk for more information.

● **Look out for patches of white or pale-grey, waxy-textured skin.** These are signs of frostbite. Go indoors and get immediate medical attention. (See the panel about frostbite, left.)

● **It might look silly, but pull large rubber dishwashing gloves over woollen gloves.** This will keep your woollen gloves dry.

● **Make sure your boots aren't too tight,** either because they're too small or because you've stuffed them with too many pairs of bulky socks. You won't have enough blood circulating to your feet and they'll get even colder. Wool or polypropylene socks are a good choice.

● **Dress in layers,** and ensure that your first is a shirt or long underwear made from synthetic microfibres, such as polypropylene. These drain sweat away from the body so you don't get too chilled. Avoid cotton, which gets wet and stays wet. Top your first layer with a fleecy garment, then a windproof jacket.

● **Equip your car for driving in snowy conditions.** Clean the snow off the car before you start driving, make sure your windshield wipers work well, clean your headlights and, in extreme conditions, use snow tyres or chains. Stock your car boot with a shovel, tow rope, ground sheet (for fitting chains), rubber gloves, plastic ice scraper, blanket and torch.

● **If you're not in good-enough shape to shovel,** pay someone else to do it for you. Shovelling snow is very strenuous. Think twice before doing it if you have a history of heart disease, heart attack or high blood pressure.

● **Stretch for 5 minutes and walk outside for 5 to 10 minutes before you start shovelling.** Here are some more tips:
● Drink plenty of water so that you're well hydrated. Don't drink caffeine or alcohol, or use nicotine products immediately before shovelling.
● Shovel early and often. Newly fallen snow is lighter than heavily packed or partially melted snow. Starting out early allows you extra time to take breaks.
● Take your time. Never remove deep snow all at once. Shovel a layer 5 to 10cm thick, then take off another 5 to 10cm.
● Pick the right shovel. A smaller shovel will require you to lift less snow, putting less strain on your body.
● Protect your back with good technique. Stand with your feet about hip-width apart for balance, and keep the shovel close to your body. Bend from the knees, not the back, and tighten your stomach muscles as you lift. Avoid twisting movements. If you need to move the snow to one side, reposition your body so your feet face the direction in which the snow will be going. Always throw the snow in front of you, not over your shoulder.
● If you experience any shortness of breath, dizziness or chest discomfort, stop immediately and seek medical attention.

WHEN COLD sets in

One of the best ways to guard against hypothermia (lowered body temperature) is to recognise the early warning signs. If someone you're with exhibits any of these, get him or her to a warm place right away. Severe cases require medical attention.
● **Shivering.** An early sign of hypothermia, shivering starts mildly, but can become more severe and finally convulsive before ceasing.
● **Slurred speech.**
● **Loss of coordination.** This might begin as difficulty tying your shoelaces or zipping your jacket, and eventually include stumbling or falling.
● **Confusion.**
● **Apathy** (for example, not caring about your own needs).
● **Irrational behaviour.**

☺ **Smear on some sunscreen and lip balm if you're out in the snow on sunny days.** And slip on a pair of sunglasses or goggles to protect your eyes from the snow's glare. A sunny day in winter is often brighter and more dangerous to your eyes than the same sun in summer, thanks to the reflection from the ice and snow.

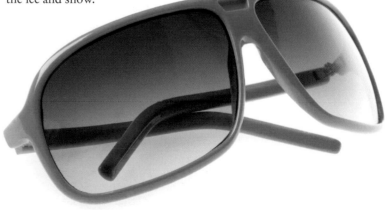

Sunglasses form a vital part of your winter wardrobe.

Index

A

abdominal and back exercises 168-76, 242, 246

abdominal crunches 174, 175, 242, 246

abdominal fat 31, 140, 213

acrylamide 239

active meditation 64-65

activity-based holidays 153

acupuncture 308

adrenaline 17, 18, 31

aerobic exercise 156, 186, 209, 263

after-dinner routine 63-67

afternoon doldrums 46-49

age-related macular degeneration (AMD) 258, 259, 260

airline food 267

air travel 280, 359-61

alarm clocks 17, 18, 73, 364

alcohol 62, 74, 119, 204, 254, 273, 310-12, 327, 361
  cutting back on 310-12
  mixed drinks 104, 118, 312
  safe limits 311

allergies 255-7, 267, 363, 366

almonds 204, 248

aloe vera 324

alpha-hydroxy acid (AHA) 326

alpha-linolenic acid 82

Alzheimer's disease 23, 301, 302, 303, 309

amaranth 95

amino acids 167, 222

ammonia 71

anger 30, 51, 208, 275, 276-80, 308

angina 31, 219

ankle weights 178

antacids 75

anthocyanins 220, 225, 261

antibiotics 217

antidepressants 266, 286

antihistamines 256

anti-inflammatories 222, 244, 245

antioxidants 21, 23, 49, 65, 66, 80, 91, 92, 222, 236, 238, 242, 259, 292, 302, 324, 325, 326

antiperspirant 337

anxiety 31, 281-4
  'worry' diary 274
  'worry time', scheduling 39

apologies 291, 292, 293

apples 22, 48, 89, 95, 102, 226, 241, 330

apricots 230

arginine 252

arm exercises 162-7

aromatherapy oils 51
  see also specific oils

aromatherapy sock 189

arthritis 163, 244, 245

artichokes 237

artificial sweeteners 102, 103, 316

artwork 40, 272

Asian pears 90

asparagus 221

aspartame 103

assertiveness skills 117, 275

asthma 110, 241, 242, 366

atherosclerosis 222

Atkins diet 96

atrial fibrillation 219

attention, paying 57, 303

aubergines 85

audio books 30, 75, 302

avocados 108, 109, 226, 228, 232, 286, 325, 327

B

backpacks 360, 366

back pain 34, 36, 138, 246, 366

back strength *see* abdominal and back exercises

bad breath 330

bagels 23, 112, 131

baked beans 103, 122

balance 184, 212

baldness 332

ball exercises 158, 170-1, 172, 174, 176, 193, 197

bananas 21, 43, 66, 75, 90, 108, 221

barley 21

basal metabolic rate 197

basil tea 274

basket organiser 19

baths 19, 75

bath soaks 324

bean burritos 122

beans 80-81, 96-97, 112, 120, 125, 128, 220, 232, 234
  see also individual varieties

bean salads 96-97, 128

beauty products 323, 324, 327

bedbugs 363

bed linen 73, 256

bedrooms 73, 74, 345-6

bedsocks 74

bedtime routine 72-75, 208
  see also sleep

beef 82, 106, 107, 117, 119, 166-7

beer 219, 225, 232, 237, 263, 267

beetroot 97, 260-1

belts 316

Benecol 22, 107, 224

bereavement 296

beta carotene 82, 89, 230, 242, 326

bicarbonate of soda 69

bike riding 149, 219, 241, 249

binge-eating disorder 314

bioplastics 79

biotin 335

biscotti 131

bladder cancer 236, 237

curtains 17, 74
custard apples 91

D

dairy products
low-fat/fat-free 204-5, 232, 236, 325
see also specific products
Danacol 22, 224
dancing 65-66, 138, 156, 158, 159-60, 178, 274
daydreaming 43
deafness 262
decision-making, times for 17
decluttering 59, 73, 208-9, 256-7
decongestants 361
deep vein thrombosis (DVT) 360
dehydration 18, 51, 207, 221, 266, 366
dementia 23, 301, 302, 303, 309
dental health 328-40
dental water jet 330
deodorant 337
depression 31, 40, 222, 249, 285-9, 309
symptoms 287
desk cleaning 47
desserts 66, 89, 102, 119, 315
dextrin 102
dextrose 103
diabetes 31, 199, 212, 238, 261, 309, 335
risk factors 31, 72, 100, 231, 287
Type 2 155, 225, 232
see also blood sugar control
diary writing 38, 66, 67, 200, 283, 291, 312, 316
dieting *see* weight, losing
difficult colleagues, dealing with 37, 38, 271, 357
dinner plates 201

dinner routine 58-62
after-dinner routine 63-67
disagreements 37, 38, 344
disappointment, coping with 282
dishwashers, cleaning 69
dish washing 245-6
disinfectants 71
dog agility classes 143
dogs 66, 74, 143, 222, 257, 275, 286, 355
domestic cleaners 148
doner kebab 123
doormats 257
drains, cleaning 69
driving 152, 222, 246, 256, 259, 296
back pain 138
car ergonomics 30
car-sharing 29
commuting 29-31
exercises while 31, 169, 178, 189
snowy conditions 370-1
drumming 288
dry-cleaning 239
dry eye syndrome 259, 260
dry skin 323, 324
dusting 69
dust mites 256

E

earplugs 75, 230, 264, 368
earwax 264
eating slowly 202, 204, 267, 274, 316
edamame 97
EGCG 237
eggs 21, 84, 99, 166, 201, 226
electric toothbrushes 329
emails 33, 37, 39, 47, 358
emergency exits 368
emollients 326, 327
empathy 279

emphysema 241
emu meat 107
endometrial cancer 237
endorphins 19, 64, 207, 282
energy, boosting 206-9
Epsom salts 324
erectile dysfunction 252
errands, running 54-57, 142-3
Escherichia coli 71
eucalyptus 75
exercise
aerobic 156, 186, 209, 263
for anxiety management 282
before bedtime 75
calisthenics 150
children and 155, 156, 158, 159
as a couple 344
gyms 50-53
heart rate recovery (HRR) 211
isometric 31, 49, 146, 167, 184
for lung power 241
for managing depression 286, 289
mental exercises 34-35
pelvic-floor exercises 169, 252
personal trainers/fitness instructors 53
progressive muscle relaxation 61, 234, 275
for stress management 273-4
stretching exercises 17, 134-9, 172, 173, 188, 209
videos and DVDs 51
weight-bearing 249, 250
and weight loss 198, 203
while driving 31, 169, 178, 189
while flying 360-1
while watching TV 52, 138, 164, 169, 172, 184, 189
at work 37, 38, 45, 48, 49, 166, 178, 186
see also strength-training; walking

monounsaturated fats 105, 107, 108, 109, 225, 234, 256, 323
morning calendar 19
morning time 66-67, 152
  exercises 135-6, 178, 188
  rituals 271-2
  wake-up routine 16-19, 148-9
motivation 17, 37, 40, 53
mould growth 69, 256, 257
mouth cancer 237, 238
mouthwash 17, 329
mozzarella cheese 106, 109
'mud room' 295
muesli 22, 62
muffins 131
multiple sclerosis 238
multi-tasking 37, 303
multivitamins 17, 211, 237, 286, 301, 324
muscle rubs 75
muscles
massaging 191
  see also strength-training
mushrooms 82
music 18, 30, 31, 38, 40, 144, 254, 275, 303, 316, 346
mustard 122
myeloma 237

N

naans 120
nail care 65, 213, 216, 334-5
nail polish 335
nail polish removers 335
napping 43, 207
neck pain 185, 186
neck pillows 73-74, 361
neck and shoulder exercises 185-9
needlework 271
neighbours 56, 57, 354, 355
news programmes 31, 208, 283, 319
night eating syndrome 61

night vision 260
noise exposure 264, 303
non-Hodgkin's lymphoma 237, 238
non-stick pans 107
'no', saying 208, 291
nose, blowing/wiping 41, 217, 267
nuts 48, 100, 108, 220, 292, 308, 314

O

oat scrub 326
oats, oatmeal 21, 23, 96, 225, 324, 326
obesity 101, 110
  childhood 155
  health-related problems 199, 242, 302
obstacle courses 160
oesophageal cancer 237
oestrogen 239, 250
oleic acid 256
olive oil 96, 99, 107, 108, 225, 236, 238, 256, 323, 325, 335, 338
olives 109, 112, 200, 325
omega-3 fatty acids 21, 108, 220, 226, 241, 246, 259-60, 286, 301, 325
omega-6 fatty acids 108, 259-60
omelettes 62, 166, 201
onions 238, 259
oral cancer 329
orange juice 23, 82, 221, 224, 230, 324
oranges 92, 221, 256
organic produce 80
organochlorines 69
osteocalcin 249
osteoporosis 47, 101, 110, 149, 163, 212, 238, 247, 250
ostrich meat 107

ovarian cancer 238
overeating 313-16
oxytocin 286
oysters 266

P

packed lunches 35, 43-45, 368
pain relief 244, 246
palm oil 108
pancreatic cancer 239
paninis 59
papayas 93
paper bags 79
parents 350-2
parking 355
Parkinson's disease 301
passion fruit 93
pasta 81, 99, 120, 234
  wholemeal 96, 99, 236
pasta salad 129, 201
pastry 119, 131
peace offerings 292
peanut butter 22, 43, 48, 108
pearl barley 96
peas 220, 221
pectin 226
pedicures 65, 337
pedometers 141, 145, 161, 200
pelvic-floor exercises 169, 252
pepper 111, 229
peppermint chocolates 40
peppermint oil 48, 65, 261, 323-4, 327, 338
PERF-ect day 211
periodontitis 328
persimmons 93
personal trainers/fitness instructors 53
perspective, keeping things in 41, 280
pesto 252
petroleum jelly 335
petroleum products 71